Registered Nurse Maternal Newborn Nursing
Care Review Module Edition 6.0

Contributors

Judith M. Wilkinson, RN, PhD, MSN, ARNP

Textbook Author
Nursing Professor
Johnson County Community College
Overland Park, Kansas

Karen Wambach, RN, PhD

Associate Professor of Nursing
University of Kansas
Kansas City, Missouri

Shirley Sherrick-Escamilla, RNC, MSN

University of Detroit Mercy
McAuley School of Nursing
Detroit, Michigan

Nancy Watts, RN, MN, PNC

CNS Maternal/Newborn Care
London Health Sciences Centre
London, Ontario

Editor-in-Chief

Leslie Schaaf Treas, RN, PhD(c), MSN, CNNP

Director of Research and Development
Assessment Technologies Institute™, LLC
Overland Park, Kansas

Editor

Jim Hauschildt, RN, EdD, MA

Director of Product Development
Assessment Technologies Institute™, LLC
Overland Park, Kansas

Copyright Notice

Important Notice to the Reader of this Publication

Assessment Technologies Institute™, LLC is the publisher of this publication. The publisher reserves the right to modify, change, or update the content of this publication at any time. The content of this publication, such as text, graphics, images, information obtained from the publisher's licensors, and other material contained in this publication are for informational purposes only. The content is not providing medical advice, and is not intended to be a substitute for professional medical advice, diagnosis, or treatment. Always seek the advice of your primary care provider or other qualified health provider with any questions you may have regarding a medical condition. Never disregard professional medical advice or delay in seeking it because of something you have read in this publication. If you think you may have a medical emergency, call your primary care provider or 911 immediately.

The publisher does not recommend or endorse any specific tests, primary care providers, products, procedures, processes, opinions, or other information that may be mentioned in this publication. Reliance on any information provided by the publisher, the publisher's employees, or others contributing to the content at the invitation of the publisher, is solely at your own risk. Healthcare professionals need to use their own clinical judgment in interpreting the content of this publication, and details such as medications, dosages or laboratory tests and results should always be confirmed with other resources.†

This publication may contain health or medical-related materials that are sexually explicit. If you find these materials offensive, you may not want to use this publication.

The publishers, editors, advisors, and reviewers make no representations or warranties of any kind or nature, including, but not limited to, the accuracy, reliability, completeness, currentness, timeliness, or the warranties of fitness for a particular purpose or merchantability, nor are any such representations implied with respect to the content herein (with such content to include text and graphics), and the publishers, editors, advisors, and reviewers take no responsibility with respect to such content. The publishers, editors, advisors, and reviewers shall not be liable for any actual, incidental, special, consequential, punitive or exemplary damages (or any other type of damages) resulting, in whole or in part, from the reader's use of, or reliance upon, such content.

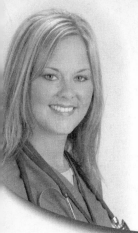

"The review modules are so helpful because they give me bulleted highlights and concise, nursing information... To top it off, you also get critical thinking exercises! These books are fantastic! They have undoubtedly been the greatest review item I have found."

Kimberly Montgomery
Nursing student

Terim Richards *Nursing student*

"I immediately went to my nurse manager after I failed the NCLEX® and she referred me to ATI. I was able to discover the areas I was weak in, and focused on those areas in the review modules and online assessments. I was much more prepared the second time around!"

Molly Obetz *Nursing student*

"The ATI review books were very helpful in preparing me for the NCLEX®. I really utilized the review summaries and the critical thinking exercises at the end of each chapter. It was nice to review the key points in the areas I was weak in and not have to read the entire book."

Lindsey Koeble *Nursing student*

"I attribute my success totally to ATI. That is the one thing I used between my first and second attempt at the NCLEX®....with ATI I passed!"

Danielle Platt *Nurse Manager • Children's Mercy Hospital • Kansas City, MO*

"The year our hospital did not use the ATI program, we experienced a 15% decrease in the NCLEX® pass rates. We reinstated the ATI program the following year and had a 90% success rate."

"As a manager, I have witnessed graduate nurses fail the NCLEX® and the devastating effects it has on their morale. Once the nurses started using ATI, it was amazing to see the confidence they had in themselves and their ability to go forward and take the NCLEX® exam."

Mary Moss *Associate Dean of Nursing and Health Programs • Mid-State Technical College • Rapids, WI*

"I like that ATI lets students know what to expect from the NCLEX®, helps them plan their study time and tells them what to do in the days and weeks before the exam. It is different from most of the NCLEX® review books on the market."

Introduction to Assessment–Driven Review

To prepare candidates for the licensure exam, many different methods have been used. Assessment Technologies Institute™, LLC, (ATI) offers Assessment–Driven Review™ (ADR), a newer approach for customized board review based on candidate performance on a series of content-based assessments.

The ADR method is a four-part process that serves as a type of competency-assessment for preparation for the NCLEX-RN®. The goal is to increase preparedness and subsequent pass rate on the licensure exam. Used as a comprehensive program, the ADR is designed to help learners focus their review and remediation efforts, thereby increasing their confidence and familiarity with the NCLEX-RN® content. This type of program identifies learners at risk for failure in the early stages of nursing education and provides a path for prescriptive learning prior to the licensure examination.

The ADR approach may be preferable to a traditional "crash course" style of review for a variety of reasons. Time restriction is a fundamental barrier to comprehensive review. Because of the difficulty in keeping up with the expansiveness of information available today, a more efficient and directed approach is needed. Individualized review that starts with the areas of deficit helps the learner narrow the focus and begin customized remediation instead of a blanket A-to-Z approach. Additionally, review that occurs sequentially over time may be preferable to after-the-fact efforts after completion of a program when faculty are no longer available to assist with remediation.

Early identification of content weaknesses may prove advantageous to progressive program success. "Smaller bites" for content achievement and a shortened lapse of time between the introduction of course content and remediation efforts is likely to be more effective in catching the struggling learner before it is too late. Regular feedback keeps learners "on track" and reduce attrition rate by identifying the learner who is "slipping." This approach provides the opportunity to tutor or implement intensified instruction before the learner reaches a point of no return and drops out of the program.

Step I: Proctored Assessment

The ADR program is a method using a prescriptive learning strategy that begins with a proctored, diagnostic assessment of the learner's mastery of nursing content. The topics covered within the ADR program are based on the current NCLEX-RN® Test Plan. Proctored assessments are administered in paper-pencil and online formats. Scores are reported instantly with Internet testing or within 24 hours for paper-pencil testing. Individual performance profiles list areas of deficiencies and guide the learner's review and remediation of the missed topics. This road map serves as a starting point for self-directed study for NCLEX® success. Learners receive a cumulative Report Card showing scores from all assessments taken throughout the program—beginning to end. Like reading a transcript, the learner and educator can monitor the sequential progress, step-by-step, an assessment at a time.

Step II: Modular Reviews

A good test is one that supports teaching and learning. The score report identifies areas of content mastery as well as a means for correction and improvement of weak content areas. Eight review modules contain concise summaries of topics with a clinical overview, therapeutic nursing management, and client teaching. Key concepts are provided to streamline the study process. The ATI modules are not intended to serve as a primary teaching source. Instead, they are designed to summarize the material relevant to the licensure exam and entry-level practice.

Learners are taught to integrate holistic care with a critical thinking approach into the review material to promote clinical application of course content. The learner constructs responses to open-ended questions to stimulate higher-order thinking. The learner may provide rationales for actions in various clinical scenarios and generate explanations of why the solution may be effective in similar clinical situations. These exercises serve as the venue to shift from traditional didactic memorization of facts toward the use of analytical and evaluative reason in a client-related situation. The clinical application scenarios involve the learner actively in the problem-solving process and stimulate an attitude of inquiry.

These exercises are designed to provoke creative problem solving for the individual learner as well as collaborative dialogue for groups of learners in the classroom. Through group discussion, learners discover the technique of elaboration. Learners use group dialogue to increase their understanding of nursing content. In study groups, they may pose questions to their peers or explain various topics in their own words, adding personal experiences with clients and examples from previously acquired knowledge of the topic. Together they learn to reframe problems and assemble evidence to support conclusions. Through the integration of multiple perspectives and the synergy involved in the exchange of ideas, this approach may also facilitate the development of effective working relationships and patterns for lifelong learning. Critical thinking exercises for each topic area situate instruction into a problem-solving environment that can capture learners' attention, increase motivation to learn, and frame the content into an application context. Additionally, the group involvement can model the process for effective team interaction.

Step III: Non-Proctored Assessments

The third step is the use of online assessments that allow users to test from any site with an Internet connection. This online battery identifies specific areas of content weakness for further directed study. The interactive style provides the learner with immediate feedback on all response options. Rationales provide additional information about the correctness of an answer to supplement learners' understanding of the concept. Detailed explanations are provided for each incorrect response to clarify topics that learners often confuse, misunderstand, or fail to remember. Readiness to learn is often peaked when errors are uncovered; thus, immediate feedback is provided when learners are most motivated to find the answer. A Performance Profile summarizes learners' mastery of content. Question descriptors for each missed item are used to stimulate inquiry and further exploration of the topic. The online assessment is intended to extend the learners' preparation for NCLEX® in a way that is personally suited to their deficiencies.

Step IV: ATI-PLAN™ DVD Series

This 12-disk set contains more than 28 hours of nursing review material. The DVD content is designed to complement ATI's Content Mastery Series™ review modules and online assessments. Using the ATI-PLAN™ navigational points, learners can easily find the content areas they want to review.

Recognizing that individuals process information in a variety of ways, ATI developed the ATI-PLAN™ DVD series to offer nursing review in a way that simulates the classroom.

However, individuals viewing the ATI-PLAN™ DVDs can navigate through more than 28 hours of material to their topics of choice. Nursing review is available at the convenience of the learner and can be replayed as often as necessary to ensure mastery of content.

The regulation of personal learning goals and the ability to plan and pursue academic intentions are the keys to successful learning. The expert teacher is the one who can determine individual learning needs and appropriate strategies to master learning. The ADR program is an efficient method of helping students prepare for the nursing licensure exam using frequent and systematic content review directed by the identified areas of content weakness. The interactive approach for mastery of nursing content focused in the areas of greatest need is likely to increase student success on the licensure exam.

ATI's ADR method parallels the nursing process in concept and in design. Both provide a framework for solving actual and potential problems purposefully and methodically. Assessment ADR-style is accomplished with ATI's battery of proctored assessments. Diagnosis is facilitated by the individual and group score reports the proctored assessments generate. Planning for improving performance in identified areas of weakness incorporates ATI's modular review system. Implementation begins with modular review and culminates in use of ATI's online assessments to validate improvement. Evaluation is reflected in the score reports, and performance can then be strengthened or further improved with the ATI-PLAN™ DVD series. Just like the nursing process, ATI's ADR prescriptive learning method often leads to specific, measurable results and highly desirable outcomes.

Table of Contents

Sociocultural Considerations

Key Points

- Family-centered care is based on the principle that families can make decisions about health care if they have adequate information.
- To provide culturally-competent care, nurses must examine their own culture and beliefs as well as become familiar with cultural values and customs different from their own.
- To provide holistic family-centered care, nurses must be knowledgeable about legal and ethical implications of situations their childbearing clients confront.
- **Key Terms/Concepts**: Family-centered care, family structure, family function, and cultural diversity

Overview

During pregnancy and childbirth, sociocultural factors impact the client's experience. Two particularly important factors are family-centered maternity care and the influence of culture on nursing care and on the client's expectations and behaviors. Open-ended questions and active listening can help the nurse support the patient's decisions regarding her health care choices.

Social Factors

- Support systems
- Income level
- Environmental factors
- Geographical location (access to care)

Principles of Family-Centered Care

Family-centered care is defined as a dynamic process of providing safe, skilled and individualized care that responds to the physical, emotional and psycho-social needs of the woman and her family. Pregnancy and birth are considered normal, healthy life events and family-centered maternity and newborn care recognizes the significance of family support and participation.

- The goal of family-centered care is to foster family unity while maintaining physical safety.
- Childbirth is a normal, healthy event.
- Childbirth affects the entire family.
- With information and professional support, families are capable of making decisions about their care.

- Core concepts include: respect, strengths, choice, information, support, flexibility, collaboration and empowerment.
- Family: A unit of two or more persons, united over a period of time, which lends both physical and emotional support

Family Types

- Adoptive
- Blended
- Cohabiting
- Communal
- Extended/multi-generational
- Nuclear
- Same sex
- Single parent
- Step-parent/family
- Traditional

Definitions

Culture: The beliefs, values, and history that are shared by a particular group and transmitted from generation to generation. Western (United States) cultural values include: democracy, individualism, cleanliness, reliance on technology, belief that health is a right, and admiration of financial success.

Ethnicity: Belonging to a particular group that shares race, language or dialect, religion, traditions, and symbols

Ethnocentrism: The belief that one's own cultural values and behaviors are superior to those of other groups

Moral: Relating to duty or obligation; pertaining to those intentions and actions of which right and wrong, virtue and vice, are predicated, or to the rules by which such intentions and actions ought to be directed; relating to the practice, manners, or conduct of men as social beings in relation to each other, as respects right and wrong, so far as they are properly subject to rules

Ethical: The philosophy or code pertaining to what is ideal in human character and conduct

Legal: A rule of conduct or action prescribed or formally recognized as binding or enforced by a controlling authority

Critical Thinking Exercise: Sociocultural Considerations

Situation: Keysha and her partner, Kevin, are Native Americans expecting their first baby's birth in approximately eight weeks. They have come to the pre-admission clinic to discuss their plans for labor and birth. As the nurse in the clinic, you describe and discuss some of the options for labor and birth that are available to them. It is their wish to have several family members present at the time of birth and to burn sweet grass during labor.

Using the concepts of family-centered care, connect with arrows or lines the care planning and interventions that the nurse may include to the correct concept(s) of family-centered care (more than one may apply).

Concept	Care Planning and Interventions
Choice	Discuss choices for labor regarding pain management and people present.
Collaboration	Discuss the role of the support person with this couple and provide information on what might be helpful in labor.
Empowerment	Encourage this couple to think about all of their options and to be comfortable choosing different ones depending on how they work in labor.
Flexibility	Encourage this family to build on their support by having family members present and including them when teaching is done.
Information	Encourage this family to continue with their traditions by the use of their sweet grass ceremony at birth.
Respect	Involve this couple in the birth planning by documenting their wishes and communicating them to the birthing unit staff.
Strengths	Prepare the birthing unit staff for their request, determine any safety and fire precautions that need to be put in place.
Support	Provide information about the hospital's birthing unit, number of family members encouraged to be present, how others might be accommodated and how their wishes regarding birth may be accommodated.

Client Teaching

Key Points

- Professional organizations have developed standards for assessing and documenting learning needs.
- Much of the nurse's teaching is spontaneous and informal, but formal teaching is also done.
- Client teaching should be based on principles of teaching and learning for adult learners.
- Client/family teaching begins in the antepartum and continues throughout the pregnancy, birth, and postpartum periods.

Overview

Client teaching is an increasingly important nursing intervention, especially the teaching of self-care. Teaching can be informal or formal. The nurse imparts knowledge and skills through discussion and demonstration. Client/family teaching begins in the antepartum and continues throughout the pregnancy, birth, and postpartum periods. Assessment of learning needs should always be done before beginning to give information.

Principles of Teaching and Learning

- Active participation increases learning.
- Learning depends on readiness of the client.
- People learn best if they think the content is important to them.
- Repetition increases retention and confidence.
- Praise and positive feedback are good motivators.
- Role modeling is an effective teaching method.
- Simple material should be presented first; progress to more complex concepts.
- Use a variety of methods.
- Present material in small amounts, not all at once.
- Follow-up is important.

Teaching Topics

- Danger signs during pregnancy
- Childbirth preparation
- Newborn care
- Postpartum self-care

- Birth control
- Nutrition during and after pregnancy
- Expected body and emotional changes
- Dealing with discomforts of pregnancy

Critical Thinking Exercise: Client Teaching

Situation: Health promotion regarding postpartum depression is a current focus in maternal/child nursing as a result of research that has shown that the incidence is much higher than was previously thought. The time that a postpartum woman and her family spend in the hospital is very short. How and when might you teach about postpartum depression to ensure that each woman and her family have enough information about this important health concern?

1. When?

2. How?

3. What adult learning principles would be utilized with this teaching plan?

4. How would you evaluate your teaching with a family?

5. What if a couple or woman/family member had a language barrier, e.g. first language is Spanish?

Medication Administration

Key Points

- Most medications cross the placenta and are delivered to the fetus.
- Medications given in pregnancy can be harmful to the fetus.
- Teach pregnant women to obtain approval from their primary care provider before taking any medication, including over-the-counter medication.
- The need for pain control in labor must be balanced with potential effects on the fetus.
- Vitamin K and erythromycin are given to newborns to prevent bleeding and ophthalmia neonatorum, respectively.

Overview

Medication administration during pregnancy and birth events includes particular attention to safe administration during pregnancy, pain control during labor and the postpartum period, and administration of medications to newborns.

Medication Administration During Pregnancy

- Most medications cross the placental barrier.
- Teach client to seek primary care provider's approval prior to any medication.
- Give medications in the lowest effective doses to minimize effects on the fetus.
- Discontinue medications as soon as possible.
- Special care is necessary in the first trimester because of fetal vulnerability during that time.
- Teratogenic agents are substances or drugs ingested by a pregnant woman that cause fetal abnormalities.
- Provide Rh-immune globulin IM at 28 weeks if mother is Rh negative, and father is Rh positive.

Medication Administration for Pain Control During Labor

- Pain medication in labor can assist a client to maintain control and actively participate in the birth experience.
- Dosage ordered is just enough to "take the edge off."
- Pain relief using:
  - Analgesics (Morphine, Demerol, Sublimaze, Nubain)—reduce pain perception
  - Barbiturates (Seconal, Nembutal, Luminal)—sedatives; rarely used

- Ataractics (Sparine, Phenergan, Vistaril)—tranquilizers
- Regional anesthesia—causes loss of sensation but not consciousness (epidural, spinal, caudal)
- All forms of pain medication cross the placental barrier.
- Herbal remedies are used in some cultures.

Medication Administration to Newborns

- Methods
  - Medicine dropper
  - Injections: Vitamin K at birth (given in vastus lateralis)
  - Ointments: Erythromycin (Ilotycin) prophylaxis to eyes
  - Administer slowly to allow infant to swallow between sips
- Client teaching
  - Vitamin A, C, and D provide supplements for bottle-fed infants
  - Acetaminophen (Tylenol)
  - Care of droppers/syringes
  - Drop into side of infant's mouth

Medications During the Postpartum Period

- Oxytocics—(oxytocin, Ergotrate, prostaglandins) to prevent postpartum bleeding
- Rh-immune globulin after delivery if mother is Rh negative, and father is Rh positive
- Analgesics
  - Combination narcotic-nonnarcotic drugs, such as acetaminophen + codeine (Tylenol #3) and oxycodone + acetaminophen (Percocet) for episiotomy pain
  - Nonsteroidal anti-inflammatory (NSAIDs), such as ibuprofen (Advil) and naproxen (Anaprox) for afterpains

Critical Thinking Exercise: Medication Administration

1. Ms. S., a G3 TPAL 2002 woman, has indicated in a birth plan that she hopes to use comfort measures during her labor and birth. However, the physician has determined that she needs augmentation for her labor based on her lack of progress. What information would you include in describing the potential side effects and benefits of oxytocin to augment labor?

2. She finds the contractions to be frequent and strong and requests information about an epidural. She is 4 cm dilated, 100% effaced and is thinking that it might be helpful. What risks and benefits would you describe to Ms. S.?

3. Her labor progresses rapidly once the oxytocin has been started and an epidural is inserted. Post birth, she has strong after-pains when her baby is breastfeeding. What information would you provide Ms. S. for pain relief (include pharmacologic strategies as well as comfort measures)?

Menstrual (Reproductive) Cycle

Key Points

- The average menstrual cycle is 28 days; flow typically lasts 4-7 days.
- Recurring anterior pituitary and ovarian hormone fluctuations cause the buildup and shedding of the endometrium.
- Menstruation ceases during pregnancy.
- **Key Terms/Concepts**: Endometrium, menstrual cycle, premenstrual syndrome (PMS), dysmenorrhea, amenorrhea

Overview

In the sexually mature female, the menstrual cycle is the periodically-recurring change in hormonal status that prepares the body for pregnancy. Anterior-pituitary and ovarian hormones cause the buildup and shedding of the endometrium (lining of the uterus). Length of menstrual cycle is determined by counting from the first day of the last menstrual bleeding to the first day of the next menstruation. In a regular 28-day cycle, ovulation occurs 14 days after the beginning of the menstrual flow. The menstrual cycle consists of two subcycles:

- Ovarian cycle: Follicular and luteal phases. Follicle-stimulating hormone (FSH) begins the cycle, which ends in mature ovum at approximately 14 days.
- Endometrial cycle: Consists of proliferation, secretory, ischemic, and menstrual phases. It prepares the endometrium and the ovum is released.

Characteristics of Menstruation

- Average menstrual cycle is 28 days (ranges from 28-34 days)
- Flow lasts 4-7 days
- Variable discomfort: "cramps," tenderness of breasts, fatigue

Therapeutic Nursing Management

- Administer mild analgesics for menstrual discomforts.
- Use a heating pad on the abdomen.
- Rest
- Exercise

Complications

- Variations in menstrual cycle due to:
    - Oral contraceptives, which decrease flow
    - Intrauterine device, which increases flow
- **Premenstrual syndrome (PMS):** A collection of symptoms preceding menstruation, characterized by headache, bloating, heaviness in lower abdomen and legs, tenderness and swelling of breasts, food cravings, depression, and irritability
- **Amenorrhea:** Cessation of menstruation; early sign of pregnancy or symptom of menopause or pathologies
- **Dysmenorrhea:** Abdominal and lower back pain during menstruation; may be accompanied by nausea and vomiting

Critical Thinking Exercise: Menstrual (Reproductive) Cycle

Situation: A teenage girl, age 15, says that her periods are "really bad." She says, "They're so unpredictable, sometimes every 24-25 days, sometimes every 32 days." They are heavy, too. I use five or six tampons a day, and I usually have cramps and pain, particularly on the first day. Is this normal?"

1. What should the nurse tell her? What self-care measures should she suggest?

2. The girl says, "I don't see how heat would help the cramps. What does it do?" What should the nurse tell her?

Conception

> ## Key Points
>
> - Fertilization usually occurs in the fallopian tube.
> - An ovum is receptive to fertilization for only 24-48 hours after ovulation.
> - Sex is determined at the moment of fertilization.
> - **Key Terms/Concepts**: Chromosome, conception, fallopian tube, fertilization, gestation, implantation, ovum, sperm, zygote

Overview

Conception is the fertilization of the female ovum by the male sperm. Fertilization occurs when a sperm enters the ovum and their nuclei unite. The ovum is receptive to fertilization for 24-48 hours after release from the ovary. Sperm are viable for 24-72 hours after ejaculation. Fertilization usually occurs in the outer third of the fallopian tube. High estrogen levels during ovulation increase peristalsis in the tube to move the zygote toward the uterus. It takes at least three days for the zygote to reach the uterine cavity.

The sex of the zygote is determined at the moment of fertilization. A mature ovum has only an X chromosome to contribute to the new nucleus. A sperm can contribute either an X or a Y chromosome. When the sperm contributes an X, the zygote is female; when the sperm contributes a Y, the zygote is male.

Cellular Multiplication: Occurs as the zygote moves through the fallopian tube toward the uterus. The zygote rapidly divides into more cells. By the time it enters the uterus it is in the form of a solid ball of 12-16 cells, called the morula.

Implantation: Occurs about one week after fertilization when the embryo buries itself in the upper segment of the uterine lining

Pregnancy: The period of time between conception and birth during which a fertilized ovum matures and grows in the female's uterus. The length of pregnancy following conception is referred to as gestation and lasts approximately 280 days (40 weeks).

Critical Thinking Exercise: Conception

Situation: A woman tells the nurse that she plans to use natural family planning (no contraceptives). She says that she knows how to recognize that ovulation has occurred. The nurse asks for clarity and the woman states that she has an increase in vaginal discharge in the middle of her cycle and that the mucous is "thin and slippery" at this time.

1. Is this a normal sign of ovulation?

2. What other signs of ovulation could the woman be taught if she wishes to use natural family planning?

Situation: A newly pregnant woman remarks, "My mother says I have to eat lots of meat if I want this baby to be a boy. Do you know of anything else that I can do to help? My husband says he does not want a wife who cannot give him sons, and I'm afraid to disappoint him."

3. How accurate is this woman's understanding of reproductive physiology? What information does she need before she can begin coping and making informed decisions about her situation?

Fetal Development

> ### Key Points
>
> - The embryonic period of fetal development is most critical because all main organ systems are developing during that time.
> - A healthy diet, moderate exercise, and adequate rest are essential, particularly during the first trimester.
> - Alcohol or drug use during the first trimester can cause greatest harm because of the organ development.
> - **Key Terms/Concepts**: Blastocyst, embryo, fetus, ectoderm, mesoderm, endoderm, ductus venosus, foramen ovale, ductus arteriosus

Overview

Fetal development is the process by which the fertilized ovum grows to maturity as a newborn. There are three periods of fetal development: the pre-embryonic period (fertilization through the first two weeks), the embryonic period (third through eighth week), and the fetal period (the eighth week though the fortieth week or birth). The embryonic period is the most critical because all main organ systems are being developed during that time. After two to three weeks of pregnancy the blastocyst differentiates to three primary germ cell layers: ectoderm, mesoderm and endoderm.

- Ectoderm: Skin, nervous system, etc.
- Mesoderm: Muscles, circulatory system, bones, reproductive system, connective tissue, etc.
- Endoderm: Alimentary and respiratory tracts, liver, bladder, and pancreas

Supportive Structures Develop Concurrently

- Placenta
- Fetal membranes
- Amniotic fluid
- Umbilical cord

Fetal Circulation

Adapted to intrauterine environment by temporary structures. The fetus receives oxygen and excretes wastes via one umbilical vein and two umbilical arteries. Fetal circulation is adapted to intrauterine environment.

Ductus Venosus: Major blood channel developing from the left umbilical vein to the inferior vena cava

Ductus Arteriosus: A fetal blood vessel that joins the aorta and pulmonary artery

Foramen Ovale: The septal opening in the fetal heart providing blood flow between the atria

The changes necessary for transition to neonatal circulation occur within the first few minutes after birth; these changes are stimulated to begin with the cutting of the umbilical cord. Blood then begins to flow through the newborn's lungs and liver. Persistent fetal circulation (PFC) is also known as persistent pulmonary hypertension of the newborn (PPHN). This condition may be life-threatening because poorly oxygenated blood is circulated to the organs and cells, resulting in acidosis. Intensive care measures, including ventilation and medication to stabilize blood pressure, are necessary to support life. The nurse's role is to provide physical care to the infant and supportive care and education to the family.

Critical Thinking Exercise: Fetal Development

Situation: J.M. is in her third trimester of pregnancy. She has been given ampicillin for a kidney infection, and is very worried about the possible effects on the fetus. She says, "What if it causes a defect in the baby's heart, or kidneys, or something?"

1. Without even knowing anything specific about the medication J.M. is taking, how realistic are her fears? What can the nurse tell her about fetal development that may help to decrease her fears?

Normal Physiological Changes of Pregnancy

Key Points

- Someone other than the mother can detect positive signs of pregnancy. They include auscultation of fetal heart tones, palpation of fetal movement, and visualization of a fetus on ultrasound.

- Most of the physiological changes of pregnancy occur as a result of shifts in the following hormone levels: Human chorionic gonadotropin (HCG), estrogen, progesterone, human placental lactogen (HPL), and relaxin.

- Except for HCG, the placenta produces all of the preceding hormones during pregnancy.

- Increased progesterone levels cause relaxation of all smooth muscles, including those in the uterus, bladder, and peripheral blood vessels.

- Major physiologic changes include (but are not limited to) the following:
  - Reproductive system: All organs become more vascular and congested.
  - Ovulation stops.
  - Cardiovascular system: Cardiac output increases dramatically; blood volume increases 1200-1600 mL above prepregnant values.
  - Gastrointestinal system: Progesterone causes relaxation of the cardiac sphincter, resulting in gastroesophageal reflux. Constipation occurs during pregnancy due to the effect of rising progesterone levels on bowel motility.
  - Urinary system: Frequency, stasis, and increased renal blood flow
  - Endocrine system: Decreased sensitivity to insulin; pituitary secretes oxytocin and prolactin

- **Key Terms/Concepts**: Gravida, para, primigravida, primipara, nulligravida, nullipara, multigravida, multipara, Goodell's sign, Chadwick's sign, quickening, and Braxton Hicks contractions

Overview

During pregnancy, the female's body undergoes significant changes. Most of the changes are influenced by shifts in the following hormone levels (these are placental hormones):

Human chorionic gonadotropin (HCG): Secreted by the trophoblastic cells during early pregnancy, it stimulates corpus luteum to produce progesterone and estrogen until the placenta can assume that function.

Estrogen: Produced by the ovaries during menstrual cycle and by the corpus luteum in early pregnancy, the placenta assumes production after the sixth or seventh week. Level remains high throughout pregnancy.

Progesterone: Produced by the corpus luteum and then by the placenta, high levels are found during pregnancy. It is the most important hormone of pregnancy because it maintains the endometrium and prevents abortion by relaxing uterine muscles. It relaxes all smooth muscles.

Human placental lactogen: Increases availability of glucose for the fetus. Its level increases steadily throughout pregnancy.

Relaxin: Inhibits uterine activity, softens connective tissue, and relaxes pelvic joints.

At the first prenatal visit, the "due date" is calculated. The estimated date of confinement (EDC), or estimated date of delivery (EDD) is calculated using Naegele's rule.

Naegele's Rule

Naegele's Rule is used to calculate the due date. This method is based on the woman's menstrual cycle. To determine the EDC, identify the first day of the last menstrual period. Subtract three months from this date. Then, add seven days to arrive at the EDC. If the pregnancy occurs in one calendar year and extends into the next, then the year change must be considered in the due date. Naegele's Rule is accurate only when the cycle is 28 days in duration with ovulation occurring at day 14.

Documentation of Pregnancy History—Common Terms

Gravida: Refers to a woman who is or has been pregnant

Para: Indicates the number of pregnancies that reached viability (20 weeks)

Primi: First

Multi: More than one

Nulli: None or never

Primigravida: A woman pregnant for the first time

Multigravida: A pregnant woman who has been pregnant before

Nulligravida: A woman who has never been pregnant

Primipara: A woman who has delivered one potentially viable fetus

Multipara: A woman who has delivered more than one potentially viable fetus

Nullipara: A woman who has not carried a fetus to viability

Shorthand Method: GTPALM (TPAL is a comprehensive system for classifying pregnancy status.)

G = gravida

T = term pregnancies

P = premature births (20-37 weeks)

A = abortions (spontaneous or induced)

L = number of living children

M = multiple gestations and births

Signs of Pregnancy

Presumptive signs are those that suggest, but do not positively indicate, pregnancy.

- Amenorrhea—absence of menstruation
- Nausea/vomiting—associated with metabolic and hormonal changes
- Breast changes—enlargement, tingling of breasts, increased sensitivity to touch, darkening of nipples and areola
- Urinary frequency—due to pressure on bladder from uterine enlargement
- Fatigue—due to increased metabolism
- Goodell's Sign—softening of a normally-firm cervix

Probable signs are strong indicators of pregnancy, short of confirmation. Two or more of these signs are highly suggestive of pregnancy. They may be detected at about the 12th week.

- Pigmentation changes—on abdomen (linea nigra) and face (chloasma gravidarum)
- Abdominal enlargement—as uterus rises out of the pelvis (12 weeks)
- Chadwick's Sign—purplish tinge of the vulva and vagina
- Hegar's Sign—softening of the lower uterine segment
- Ballottement—detection of fetus floating in amniotic fluid
- Braxton Hicks contractions—irregular, painless uterine contraction
- Palpation of fetal outline—by external examiner at 26-28 weeks
- Quickening—fluttering sensation felt by pregnant women when fetus moves (16-20 weeks)
- Positive pregnancy test—Maternal blood or urine test for human chorionic gonadotropin (HCG). Can be performed as early as 8-10 days after conception

Positive signs

- Detection of fetal heart tones
- Palpation of fetal movement
- Ultrasonic evidence of a fetus

Physiological Changes of Pregnancy

Reproductive system

- Uterus—enlarges; irregular, painless contractions occur
- Ovaries—ovulation stops due to high levels of placental estrogen and progesterone
- Vagina—becomes softer, mucosa thickens, vascularity increases, vaginal discharge increases and becomes more acidic
- Breasts—increase in size and become full and tender; areola darken; colostrum is excreted
- Cervix—softens (Goodell's sign), becomes congested with blood (Chadwick's sign), proliferating glands form mucus plug

Musculoskeletal system

- Relaxation of joints

- Widening of symphysis pubis
- Waddling gait
- Lordosis
- Increased back strain

Cardiovascular system

- Heart muscle enlarges.
- Heart rotates upward and to the left.
- Stroke volume increases.
- Cardiac output increases, primarily as a result of expanded vascular volume.
- Pulse rate increases by about 10-15 beats per minute.
- Peripheral vascular resistance falls under the influence of progesterone and prostaglandins.
- Femoral venous pressure increases.
- Blood pressure remains essentially the same, despite increased blood volume.
- Blood volume increases to 1200-1600 mL above pre-pregnant values.
- Total red cell mass increases; however, the increase in plasma volume is even more pronounced, resulting in dilution of the red blood cell mass and a decline in hematocrit (this is not true anemia).
- White blood cell count increases to an average of 10,000/mm^3.
- Clotting factors increase, offering protection against bleeding, but increasing chance of thrombophlebitis.

Respiratory System

- Oxygen consumption increases by about 20 percent.
- Dyspnea is common.
- Nosebleeds and nasal stuffiness are common.
- Rib cage widens.
- Respiratory depth increases.

Gastrointestinal System: Gastrointestinal system changes are significant because they create some of the discomforts of pregnancy. Most of the changes are produced by progesterone, which relaxes the muscles of the stomach and intestines.

- Gums appear red and swollen and bleed easier, caused by elevated levels of estrogen.
- Nausea and vomiting may occur.
- Delayed gastric emptying and reduced tone of cardiac (esophageal) sphincter allows reflux of acidic stomach contents, producing heartburn.
- Decreased motility in large intestine allows more water to be absorbed; may cause constipation and hemorrhoids.
- Increased thirst and appetite.

Urinary system

- Frequent urination is common, particularly in the first and third trimesters.
- Urinary stasis predisposes to urinary tract infection.

- Renal blood flow increases.

Endocrine system

- Placenta becomes an endocrine organ and produces large amounts of estrogen, progesterone, and glucocorticoids.
- After the first trimester, the pancreas produces additional insulin; however, by the end of pregnancy, tissue sensitivity to insulin falls by up to 80 percent.
- Oxytocin and prolactin are secreted by the pituitary gland.
- Thyroid gland enlarges; basal metabolic rate increases.

Critical Thinking Exercise: Normal Physiological Changes of Pregnancy

Situation: M.P. has come to the clinic on September 10th. She states that the first day of her last menstrual period was June 10. She has performed a home pregnancy test, which was positive. She says, "I think that I may be pregnant. I've had nausea in the morning and vomiting (2-3 times/week)." M.P. tells you, as the nurse in the clinic, that she had an abortion when she was 18. She also had a miscarriage at 11 weeks last year. On examination, Chadwick and Hegar's signs are present. M.P. states that she is often tired and that for the past three months, she has experienced urinary frequency.

1. From this data, can you be sure that M.P. is pregnant? Why or why not?

2. What information do you need to confirm M.P.'s pregnancy?

3. What information would you give M.P. regarding nausea and vomiting during pregnancy?

4. What is M.P.'s due date, or estimated date of birth (EDB)?

5. Using the terms, "gravida" and "para" and the TPAL method for describing obstetrical history, describe M.P.'s GTAL. (gravida 3, para 0, TPAL: 30020)

Nutrition

Key Points

- Ideally, good nutrition should begin before a woman becomes pregnant.
- Nutrition during pregnancy affects the size of the baby and its stores of nutrients for the neonatal period.
- Folic acid supplements are recommended during pregnancy to prevent neural tube defects.
- Iron supplements are routinely prescribed to prevent anemia and assure adequate fetal stores.
- An additional intake of 300 calories a day is required during pregnancy.
- A lactating woman requires 2,700-2,800 calories per day.
- A lactating woman should consume 3,000 mL of fluids per day.
- Recommended weight gain in pregnancy is 35 lbs.
- The general pattern of weight gain is 3.5 lbs during the first trimester, and just under l lb per week during the rest of the pregnancy.
- Weight loss diets should not begin until well after the puerperium when tissue repair has been completed
- **Key Terms/Concepts**: Folic acid, iron supplement, nutrition, weight gain pattern, inadequate weight

Overview

Nutrition is the process by which a living organism assimilates and uses food. Nutrition is especially important in pregnancy because the woman's food intake must nourish her own body and that of the growing fetus. Nutrition affects the size of the baby and whether it has adequate stores of nutrients after birth. Lack of some vital nutrients (e.g., folic acid) can cause birth defects. Nutrition teaching can be based on the food guide pyramid, which includes the following groups: grains, cereals, rice, and pastas; fruits; vegetables; dairy foods; meats and other proteins; and fats, oils and sweets. Nearly all nutrient needs (calories, carbohydrates, proteins, fats, vitamins, minerals, and water) increase during pregnancy, but in most cases they can be met through the diet. Supplements of iron and folic acid are usually prescribed because it is difficult to ingest them in adequate amounts.

Weight gain during pregnancy is an important determinant of fetal growth. The recommended gain is 25 to 35 pounds for women with a normal pre-pregnant weight. However, the pattern of weight gain is as important as the total increase. The general recommendation is for about 3.5 pounds during the first trimester and just under 1 pound a week during the rest of the pregnancy.

During Pregnancy

- Increase daily intake of vitamins, minerals, and protein, (e.g., meat, fish, eggs, poultry, beans, legumes, seeds, nuts, milk, and dairy protein).
- An additional 300 calories a day are required.
- Vitamins and minerals are added via prescription.
    - Folic acid is prescribed almost routinely now to prevent neural tube defects.
    - Most practitioners prescribe iron supplements of 30 mg daily to prevent anemia and assure fetal stores are adequate.

Postpartum

- A well-balanced, 2,200-2,300 calorie diet is optimal in the postpartum period.
- High protein, vitamins, and minerals promote tissue repair.
- The lactating woman usually requires 2,700-2,800 calories per day.
- A diet high in fiber will help prevent constipation.
- At least 2,000 mL fluid /day is necessary in the postpartum period. For the lactating woman, increase to 3000 mL/day.
- Postpone weight-loss diets until well after the puerperium.

Maternal Risk Factors for Inadequate Nutrition in Pregnancy

- Abnormal pre-pregnancy weight (e.g., the woman who is underweight may not have enough money for food, or may have an eating disorder; the obese woman may not wish to gain additional weight).
- Preexisting anemia
- Unsafe eating patterns: anorexia, bulimia
- Substance abuse
- Inappropriate consumption; pica
- Smoking
- Extreme vegetarianism
- Nausea and vomiting
- Multiparity
- Adolescence
- Low socioeconomic status
- Cultural influences, which may include dietary taboos

Complications of Inadequate Nutrition

- Excessive weight gain during pregnancy
- Insufficient weight gain during pregnancy
- Anemia
- Compromised fetal development
- Low birth weight of neonate

Critical Thinking Exercise: Nutrition

Situation: C.J. is at the end of the first trimester of her pregnancy. Her normal pre-pregnant weight was 120 lbs. She now weighs 125 lbs, and she is concerned that she is "getting fat." Her food diary indicates that she is eating a fairly well balanced diet except for an insufficient intake of dairy products and iron-rich foods. She says, "I don't drink milk. I've never liked it." C.J. states that she has been taking her folic acid supplement as prescribed.

1. How would you assess C.J.'s weight gain: too much, too little, or just right?

2. With regard to C.J.'s weight, what problem should be of most concern to the nurse?

3. How should the nurse respond to C.J.'s statement that she doesn't like milk?

4. What medical complication is likely to occur if C.J.'s iron intake remains low?

5. C.J's caregiver prescribes an iron supplement. Why do you think this was necessary? Why didn't the nurse simply advise her to eat more iron-rich foods, in the same way she addressed her dairy products deficiency?

6. How would it further complicate C.J.'s nutritional status if she were a strict vegetarian?

7. How would it further complicate her nutritional status if she were a smoker?

C.J. asks specific questions to ensure that she is eating to get enough calories and nutritive value. For each of the nutrients listed below, choose two foods and the correct amount that should be in the diet of a pregnant woman:

Nutrient	Amount	Foods
Calcium	1. 15mg	8. brown bread, beef
Folic Acid	2. 1300mg	9. broccoli, strawberries
Iron	3. 30mg	10. eggs, cheese
Protein	4. 60g	11. fortified margarine, fruits
Vitamin A	5. 600ug	12. oranges, asparagus
Vitamin C	6. 70mg	13. spinach, baked beans
Zinc	7. 800ug	14. spinach, dried fruits

Nursing Management of the Client with Prenatal Danger Signs

Key Points

The danger signs that should be reported to the primary care provider are:
- Any amount and color of vaginal bleeding
- Rupture of membranes
- Severe, persistent headache
- Edema of face and hands
- Abdominal or epigastric pain
- Chills and fever
- Painful urination or flank pain
- Persistent vomiting
- Absence of fetal movement

Overview

Although pregnancy is considered to be a normal, healthy condition, complications can occur. It is important to teach the pregnant woman the difference between common discomforts of pregnancy (such as varicose veins, heartburn, and constipation) and signs of dangerous complications. Women should be taught to report the following danger signs and symptoms to the health care provider immediately.

Danger Signs

- Vaginal bleeding, whether bright red or brown, in any amount
- Rupture of membranes
- Severe, persistent headache
- Visual disturbances
- Edema of face or hands
- Abdominal pain
- Epigastric pain
- Elevated temperature (above 101° F) and chills
- Painful urination
- Persistent vomiting (over one day)
- Change in, or absence of, fetal movement (e.g., no movement for 6-8 hours)

Client Teaching

- When reporting vaginal bleeding or other fluid leakage, describe color, odor, and amount.
- Monitor urine output for amount, blood, and foul smell.
- Recognize and report signs and symptoms of pregnancy-induced hypertension: weight gain of more than five pounds since last prenatal visit, edema (face and hands), persistent headache, lightheadedness, dizziness, double/blurred vision, or epigastric pain.
- Check body temperature if other signs occur.
- Consider preterm labor if low back pain or cramping before 36 weeks.

Complications

The "danger signs" may indicate complications such as pregnancy-induced hypertension, placenta previa, premature labor, infection, and so forth. All may be associated with maternal and fetal morbidity and mortality.

Critical Thinking Exercise: Nursing Management of the Client with Prenatal Danger Signs

Situation: A pregnant woman comes to the the clinic for her regular 24-week appointment and reports some symptoms she is having. She says that she is having urinary frequency, but no burning with urination; and that her temperature is 99.1° F. She also reports that she is having a mucoid discharge from her vagina.

1. What additional assessments and history taking will the nurse do?

2. What else does the nurse need to know in order to be certain that the woman's vaginal discharge is normal?

3. This same woman returns at 28 weeks. What would be included in her teaching at this time? List three topics and at least two things that would be taught to ensure that this woman knows what to do in these situations.

Nursing Management of the Client with Hyperemesis Gravidarum

Key Points

- Mild nausea and vomiting are normal discomforts of pregnancy; they usually disappear in the third month.
- Hyperemesis gravidarum should be suspected if vomiting is persistent and uncontrollable.
- Hyperemesis gravidarum may require hospitalization for intravenous hydration and nutritional supplements.
- Severe and continued hyperemesis results in fluid and electrolyte imbalances that can compromise the fetus.

Overview

Mild nausea and vomiting are common during the early part of pregnancy (up to 70% of pregnancies). Commonly called "morning sickness," it is thought to be due to elevated progesterone, estrogen, and human chorionic gonadotropin (HCG) levels but may also be associated with a variety of other factors such as vitamin B deficiency, genetic factors, low maternal age and smoking. Symptoms may be aggravated by fatigue, cooking odors, and emotional stress. Women need reassurance that nausea and vomiting are normal and will usually disappear in the third month.

Hyperemesis gravidarum is a more serious condition that requires medical attention. Hyperemesis gravidarum begins in early pregnancy and may continue throughout the pregnancy. The cause is unknown. The highest incidence is among primigravidas, multifetal pregnancies, and women with psychiatric disorders (these may predate the condition or contribute to it). Hospitalization is recommended if symptoms cannot be controlled at home.

Signs and Symptoms of Hyperemesis Gravidarum

- Persistent, uncontrollable vomiting
- Decreased urinary output
- Rapid pulse
- Low-grade fever
- Weight loss

Diagnostic Tests and Lab

- Hematocrit, hemoglobin
- Electrolytes

- Urine protein and acetone

Therapeutic Nursing Management of Nausea and Vomiting

- Implement common nausea and vomiting nursing interventions:
  - Recommend smaller, frequent meals; include salty foods.
  - Suggest crackers before arising.
  - Avoid spicy and fried foods.
  - Advise to remain upright for 30 minutes after eating.
  - Vitamin B supplements and ginger may also be beneficial.
  - Discuss use of antacids with primary care provider.
- Treatments and goals for hospitalized client:
  - Control of vomiting
  - NPO
  - Progress to small feedings every 2-3 hours when tolerated.
  - Quiet environment
  - Intake & output
  - Adequate nutrition–nasogastric tube feeding may be necessary.

Pharmacologic Management

- Sedatives
- Antiemetics
- Correction of fluid and electrolyte imbalances
- Intravenous fluids

Complications

- Dehydration
- Electrolyte imbalance
- Severe weight loss
- Metabolic alkalosis

Critical Thinking Exercise: Nursing Management of the Client with Hyperemesis Gravidarum

Situation: K.L. has been admitted to the hospital with a diagnosis of hyperemesis gravidarum. She is in the ninth week of her pregnancy and has lost 5% of her pre-pregnant weight. She cannot tolerate oral fluids or food, and she is receiving lactated Ringer's solution intravenously (IV).

1. What nursing diagnoses would be appropriate for K.L.?

2. All of the data suggest that K.L. is at risk for Altered Nutrition. Which data specifically supports a diagnosis of actual Altered Nutrition?

3. Why is K.L. receiving intravenous fluids?

K.L. continues to be very nauseous and vomits 3-4 times a day. The gastroenterologist involved in her care recommends total parenteral nutrition (TPN) until she is able to keep oral intake down. She and her husband receive training in preparation for home care. She tells you that she is worried about the next few weeks and has even considered terminating the pregnancy.

4. As her nurse, you tell her to:?

5. What other professionals would you consider involving in K.L.'s care prior to discharge?

Nursing Management of the Client
with Pregnancy Induced Hypertension (PIH)

Key Points

- Signs of preeclampsia are: elevated blood pressure, edema of the face and hands, sudden weight gain, and 1+ to 2+ proteinuria.
- Signs of severe preeclampsia are: further increase in blood pressure, headache, blurred vision, epigastric pain, increasing proteinuria, nausea, and vomiting.
- Signs of eclampsia are seizures or coma.
- Magnesium sulfate is used to control seizures; the antidote is calcium gluconate; toxic effects include depressed reflexes, depressed respirations, oversedation, and circulatory collapse.
- PIH is a major cause of fetal and maternal death.
- Maternal death is often a result of pulmonary edema, cardiac or other organ failure, or cerebral hemorrhage.
- **Key Terms/Concepts**: Preeclampsia, eclampsia, HELLP syndrome, disseminated intravascular coagulation (DIC), proteinuria

Overview

Gestational hypertension refers to elevated blood pressure (>140/90) that develops after 20 weeks in pregnancy. It is compounded by proteinuria (+1 or greater). Edema is no longer a defining characteristic for diagnosis. Chronic hypertension is defined as increased blood pressure (>140/90 prior to 20 weeks gestation in pregnancy (Advances in Labour and Risk Management, 2000). Pregnancy-induced hypertension (PIH) occurs in 6-8% of all pregnancies and is the second-leading cause of maternal deaths. Ending the pregnancy and delivering the infant is a way to treat the disease. PIH is characterized by hypertension, edema, and proteinuria. It is serious because of the arteriolar vasoconstriction, systemic vasospasms, and vascular changes that occur. Vasospasms result in fluid volume excess, resulting in fluid retention. PIH is classified as preeclampsia or eclampsia, depending on the severity of the symptoms. Preeclampsia is characterized by hypertension with proteinuria or edema developing after 20 weeks gestation. Eclampsia is a progression of preeclampsia characterized by epigastric pain, grand mal seizures, and coma.

Risk Factors

- Family history of hypertension
- Weight extremes
- Diabetes
- Multiple pregnancy

- Inadequate prenatal care
- Previous history of PIH
- Chronic renal disease
- Rh incompatibility
- Occurrence is higher among primiparas; women who are younger than 20 or older than 35 years of age; women with chronic hypertension, diabetes mellitus, or renal failure; and women in lower socioeconomic groups

Diagnostic Tests and Lab

- Hemoglobin/hematocrit
- CBC
- Liver enzymes
- Platelets
- DIC profile, clotting studies
- Chemistry panel, including: BUN, creatinine, glucose, uric acid

Signs and Symptoms

Preeclampsia

- Blood pressure 140/90 or an increase of 30 mmHg systolic or 15 mmHg diastolic
- Edema—1+ pitting edema after being on bed rest for 12 hours
- Sudden excessive weight gain (5 or more pounds a week)
- Swelling of the feet, hands, and face that does not resolve after bed rest for 12 hours
- Proteinuria (1+ or 2+, or greater than 3g/L in 24-hour specimen)

Severe Preeclampsia

- Blood pressure of 160/110 or higher
- Extensive edema, including pulmonary
- Cyanosis
- Decreased urine output
- Continuing weight gain of more than 2 pounds/week
- Nausea and vomiting
- Headache
- Epigastric pain (sign that the disease is worsening)
- Increased hematocrit
- Proteinuria (3+ or 4+ or greater than 4g/L in 24 hours)

Eclampsia

- Seizures (grand mal) or coma (preceded by further increase in blood pressure, headache, blurred vision, epigastric pain, and nausea/vomiting)

Therapeutic Nursing Management

- Take vital signs frequently, especially blood pressure.
- Assess edema and document 1+, 2+, 3+, 4+.
- Record daily weight.
- Encourage a high-protein diet.
- Position client on left side.
- Test urine for protein/specific gravity every 8 hours.
- Measure and record intake and output.
- Assess deep tendon reflexes every 2-4 hours.
- Insert Foley catheter (as ordered).
- Implement seizure precautions.
- Assess for increasing symptoms.
- Assemble oral airway, suction, and oxygen equipment at bedside.
- Assess fetal status by FHR and fetal movement sheet.
- Ensure bed rest or restricted activity.
- Decrease environmental stimuli.
- Prepare client for non-stress tests (NST) to assess fetal well-being.
- If situation becomes critical, prepare client for immediate C-section.

Pharmacologic Management

- Magnesium sulfate (MgSO4) to control seizures
- Observe for toxicity, magnesium levels, respiratory depression, loss of reflexes, circulatory collapse, muscle weakness, over-sedation and confusion, extreme thirst, or hypotension.
- Have antidote available: calcium gluconate.

Complications

- PIH is a major cause of maternal and fetal death.
- Fetal complications of PIH include: intrauterine growth retardation (IUGR) and fetal distress caused by hypoxia.
- Maternal complications include: hemorrhage, cardiac difficulties, disseminated vascular coagulation (DIC).
- HELLP syndrome reflects severity of the disease
    - Hemolysis
    - Elevated
    - Liver enzymes
    - Low
    - Platelets
- Eclampsia is associated with an increased risk for maternal death rate related to pulmonary edema, organ failure, cardiac failure, or cerebral hemorrhage.

Critical Thinking Exercise: Nursing Management of the Client with Pregnancy–Induced Hypertension (PIH)

Situation: S.J. is a 38-year-old primigravida at 32 weeks gestation. She is a single mother, living with her parents and two sisters. She has a high-stress sales job being paid by commissions only. She admits that she doesn't "eat right." She says she doesn't have time to prepare meals and eats mostly fast foods and "junk food." Her mother does cook for the family, but the meals are high in fat and sodium. S.J. is 5 ft. 2 in. tall and her prepregnant weight was 180 lbs. S.J. has edema of the feet, ankles, and hands.

1. What risk factors does S.J. have for pregnancy-induced hypertension?

2. What vital sign is the most important for the nurse to assess at this time?

3. What should the nurse ask S.J. in order to assess her edema further?

4. S.J.'s blood pressure is 146/90. Her health problem will be managed on an outpatient basis. After being taught to check her blood pressure and to check her urine for protein, she is asked to keep a record of her weight, urine protein, B/P, and fetal movement count. What other advice should the nurse provide?

Nursing Management of the Client with Gestational Diabetes

Key Points

- Gestational diabetes is a type of diabetes mellitus. It is called "gestational" because it first occurs or is identified during pregnancy.
- Diabetes is a disorder of carbohydrate metabolism related to decreased production of or resistance to insulin.
- Pregnancy creates resistance to insulin in maternal cells; if the pancreas cannot produce enough insulin to compensate, then maternal hyperglycemia occurs.
- Gestational diabetes is usually detected by screening with a 50 gram glucose challenge test at 24-28 weeks in pregnancy or by review of risk factors such as family history of type II diabetes, previous history of gestational diabetes, >4000 gm. infant in previous pregnancy or unexplained stillbirth. It is diagnosed by an oral glucose test.
- Treatment includes diet, exercise, glucose monitoring, and evaluation of fetal status.
- If blood glucose levels cannot be maintained by diet and exercise, insulin is prescribed.
- Oral hypoglycemics are not commonly used in pregnancy.
- The major fetal complications are birth injuries (because of macrosomia) and neonatal hypoglycemia.
- Major maternal complications include hyperglycemia, dystocia, hydramnios, and an increased risk of pregnancy-induced hypertension
- **Key Terms/Concepts**: Gestational diabetes, hyperglycemia

Overview

Gestational diabetes is carbohydrate intolerance of variable severity that is first recognized during pregnancy. It may occur as a result of (a) previously existing but unidentified disease, (b) an existing metabolic problem that was being compensated, but which can no longer be compensated because of the demands of pregnancy, or (c) altered carbohydrate metabolism caused by changing hormone levels. The diagnosis is usually made in the second half of pregnancy when the fetus' nutrient demands increase. Most women with gestational diabetes are managed by diet alone, and pregnant women are routinely screened for the disease at 24-28 weeks. The first indication of gestational diabetes is usually glycosuria on the urinalysis at the first prenatal visit. The symptoms of gestational diabetes disappear in the first few weeks after delivery. Postpartum, this woman should be tested with a fasting blood sugar and given health teaching regarding her risk for development of Type

II diabetes within the next five to 10 years. Lifestyle changes such as diet and exercise would be included in this teaching, as well as, follow-up with her care provider at six weeks' time.

Risk Factors

- Previously large newborn (9 pounds or more)
- Family history of diabetes mellitus
- Glucosuria on two successive occasions
- Obesity (>200 pounds)
- Spontaneous abortions or stillbirths
- Multiparity
- Presence of hydramnios
- Previous baby with congenital anomaly
- Hypertension

Diagnostic Tests and Lab

- Fasting blood sugar (FBS)— level of 100-120 mg/dL acceptable
- Glucose challenge test
- Routine urine testing via dipstick
- Blood glucose levels, if indicated by results of urine tests

Signs and Symptoms

- Hyperglycemia on routine challenge test (24-28 weeks) where results are 140 mg/dL
- Ketoacidosis
- Classic signs of diabetes—polydipsia, polyphagia, polyuria, glycosuria

Therapeutic Nursing Management

- Provide diet instruction (strict adherence to 2,000-2,400 calorie diet).
- Teach self-care/hygiene.
- Monitor blood glucose and urine for ketones.
- Encourage exercise.
- Teach the symptoms of hypoglycemia and ketoacidosis.
- Maintain fetal surveillance, especially in third trimester: echocardiography, ultrasound, fetal movements, and non-stress test.

Pharmacologic Management

- Insulin does not cross the placenta.

Complications

- Pregnancy-induced hypertension
- Infection (e.g., urinary tract infection, postpartum infection)
- Increased incidence of stillbirth
- Spontaneous abortion
- Preterm or early labor
- Intrauterine growth retardation (IUGR)
- Macrosomia
- Hydramnios
- Fetal hypoglycemia (common)
- Maternal hypoglycemia
- Fetal congenital abnormalities (cardiac, CNS, etc.)
- C-section, forceps, or vacuum extraction for large infant
- Perinatal asphyxia
- Newborn shoulder dystocia (related to size)
- Birth trauma
- Neonatal respiratory distress
- Neonatal hypoglycemia, hypocalcemia, polycythemia, and hyperbilirubinemia

Critical Thinking Exercise: Nursing Management of the Client with Gestational Diabetes

Situation: K.C. is 34 years old. She is a gravida 2, para 0. Her first pregnancy ended in a stillbirth. At her first prenatal visit her diabetes screening was negative. However, in her second trimester, she is diagnosed with gestational diabetes. She is normal weight for her height, and her weight gain has followed the recommended pattern thus far in pregnancy.

1. What risk factors does K.C. have for gestational diabetes?

2. What test was probably used to diagnose K.C.'s diabetes?

3. Why do you think K.C.'s urine was negative for glucose on her first prenatal visit, but her glucose screening test was positive during her second trimester?

4. K.C.'s glucose tolerance test was initially >95 mg/dL (>5.3 mmol/L) and her 1 hour test was >180 mg/dL (>10.0 mmol/L). How would you interpret these results? How would you plan her care?

5. During labor her blood glucose levels may need to be monitored every 1-2 hours. How would you explain this?

6. K.C. has decided to breastfeed this baby. How would you encourage her with this process?

Nursing Management of the Client with Anemia

Key Points

- Iron requirements double during pregnancy to 30 mg/day.
- Iron is needed for maternal hemoglobin formation and for fetal stores.
- It is nearly impossible to ingest enough dietary iron to meet the iron requirements of pregnancy.
- Medical guidelines recommend that all pregnant women receive a supplement of 30 mg of ferrous iron daily, beginning at 12 weeks of gestation (pregnant women with iron deficiency anemia receive 60-120 mg daily).
- Complications of anemia include preterm birth, poor wound healing, infection, and cardiac failure during labor.

Overview

Iron deficiency anemia is the most common hematological disorder in pregnancy. Maternal blood volume increases by 1500 mL during pregnancy, so iron is needed to expand the maternal red blood cell mass. Maternal iron requirement raises significantly the last half of the pregnancy as the fetus's requirements increase. This leads to the depletion of maternal iron stores. Diet alone cannot replace gestational iron losses. Even women with good nutrition will most likely end pregnancy with an iron deficit if they do not take an iron supplement during pregnancy.

Risk Factors

- Previous pre-pregnant anemia
- Poor nutritional status
- Close spacing of pregnancies
- Twin gestations
- Excessive vaginal bleeding prior to or as a result of pregnancy

Diagnostic Tests and Lab

- Hemoglobin level
- Hematocrit level
- Nutritional history
- Serum ferritin

Signs and Symptoms

- Hemoglobin level below 10 mg/dL
- Hematocrit level below 35%
- Fatigue/pallor
- Susceptibility to infection
- Intolerance to blood loss after delivery

Therapeutic Nursing Management

- Provide education about food sources rich in iron: fortified cereals, enriched breads, liver, meat, dried fruits (e.g., raisins), leafy green vegetables, and legumes. Some women do not tolerate iron supplements well, so food sources are important.
- Instruct about the need for high fluid intake and a high-fiber diet to prevent constipation.
- Instruct about the need for supplemental iron.
- Instruct that vitamin C will increase absorption.
- Teach mother that iron will produce a black stool and may cause other gastrointestinal symptoms such as gas and nausea.
- If it can be tolerated, iron is best absorbed if taken when stomach is empty.
- Milk inhibits absorption.

Pharmacologic Management

- Oral: ferrous sulfate or ferrous gluconate
- Parenteral (if oral not tolerated): iron-dextran complex (Imferon)

Complications

- Congestive heart failure during labor
- Poor wound healing
- Increased risk for postpartum hemorrhage and infection
- Preterm birth
- Risk for small for gestational age (SGA) babies

Critical Thinking Exercise: Nursing Management of the Client with Anemia

Situation: T.C. is in the 26th week of her pregnancy. Her hemoglobin is 9.5 g/dL and her hematocrit is 30%. She says, "My sister's hemoglobin was low, too. They said it was normal, though, because your blood is 'thinner' during pregnancy. I'm glad I'm not anemic."

1. One week later, T.C. telephones to say that she has abdominal discomfort after taking her iron pill. What should the nurse advise?

2. How should the nurse respond to T.C.'s statement?

3. The care provider prescribes an oral iron supplement for T.C. The nurse tells her that she should include foods high in vitamin C (e.g., oranges, grapefruits, tomatoes, melons, and strawberries). Why?

4. The nurse also tells T.C. to avoid consuming these foods at the same time as taking the iron supplement: bran, egg yolk, oxalates (e.g., spinach), coffee, tea, and milk. She advises her to take her iron supplement between meals. Why?

5. During this same telephone call, T.C. tells the nurse that she is not constipated, but that her stools are black. What should the nurse advise?

Nursing Management of the Client with an Abortion

Key Points

- Abortion occurs when pregnancy is lost before viability (20 weeks gestation).
- Common symptoms are abdominal cramping and vaginal bleeding/spotting.
- Common complications are hemorrhage and infection.
- Nursing care includes monitoring for bleeding and providing emotional support.
- **Key Terms/Concepts:** Spontaneous abortion, induced abortion, incomplete abortion, missed abortion

Overview

Pregnancy that ends before the fetus can survive outside the uterus is called an abortion. Abortions occur in the first or second trimesters before 20 weeks gestation, and are either spontaneous or induced. Spontaneous abortion occurs naturally, without outside intervention. Miscarriage is the lay term, but it is becoming more widely used among healthcare workers because the term abortion has negative connotations for some women. Induced abortion is the intentionally-produced loss of pregnancy by a woman or others. This is also known as elective abortion.

Risk Factors

- Defects in ovum or sperm
- Inadequate intrauterine environment, defective implantation
- Maternal diseases that predispose to abortion: infection, diabetes, hormonal deficiencies, incompetent cervix
- Fetal or placental developmental defects, genetics

Diagnostic Tests and Lab

- Pregnancy test to assess HCG levels
- CBC, hematocrit, hemoglobin to assess for anemia

Signs and Symptoms

- Vaginal bleeding
- Abdominal/uterine cramping
- Low backache
- Eventual rupture of membranes and dilation of the cervix

Therapeutic Nursing Management

- Take a health history.
- Document onset, duration, amount, and character of bleeding.
- Monitor vital signs.
- Prepare for a dilation and curettage (D & C) if spontaneous abortion occurs in first trimester.
- Provide emotional support.
- Provide bed rest.
- Instruct the client to avoid intercourse until the bleeding stops.

Complications

- Incomplete abortion—when part of the products of conception are not expelled
- Missed abortion—when the fetus dies but is not expelled for 4-6 weeks after fetal loss
- Disseminated intravascular coagulation (DIC) following long duration of missed abortion
- Hemorrhage
- Infection

Critical Thinking Exercise: Nursing Management of the Client with an Abortion

Situation: A woman in the 14th week of pregnancy is admitted with a dilated cervix, severe abdominal cramping, and heavy vaginal bleeding. She is diagnosed with inevitable miscarriage (abortion).

1. What should the initial nursing assessment include, and why?

2. Based on the data provided in the situation, what nursing diagnoses can you be sure this woman has? (Write the etiologies of the diagnoses, as well.)

3. For what other nursing diagnoses should the nurse assess?

4. What expected outcomes are appropriate for this woman?

5. This woman has experienced or is experiencing a loss. How would you incorporate her partner's emotional needs in her care planning while at the hospital/clinic? What follow-up would be appropriate for this woman/partner?

Nursing Management of the Client with Exposure to Rubella

Key Points

- Rubella is a viral infection transmitted by droplets (e.g., by sneezing).
- Congenital rubella infection frequently results in congenital anomalies, deafness, and even fetal death.
- Pregnant women should not be vaccinated because of the risk of acquiring the disease.
- All pregnant women should be screened for rubella.
- A titer of 1:8 or less indicates susceptibility to infection; a titer of 1:16 indicates immunity.

Overview

Rubella, also called German measles or three-day measles, is a highly infectious disease caused by a virus, which produces a fever and rash 14-21 days after exposure. The virus enters the upper respiratory system and after seven to 10 days, enters the blood stream. The fetus is at risk if the infection occurs during the first trimester. The infection can lead to defective fetal development directly related to organ formation at the time of maternal exposure. Rubella can result in fetal blindness, hearing loss, heart disease, mental retardation, or demise. Women of childbearing age who are not pregnant should be immunized against rubella. Pregnant women should not be vaccinated because of the possibility of developing a rubella infection while pregnant.

Risk Factors

- Rubella antibodies (unimmunized)
- Children in the home (unimmunized)

Diagnostic Tests and Lab

- Screening done in early pregnancy for presence of rubella antibodies a titer of 1:16 or more indicates immunity–a titer of 1:8 indicates susceptibility to infection.
- Hemagglutination inhibition test (HAI)
- Radioimmunoassay test (RIA)

Signs and Symptoms

- Rash
- Fever
- Cold-like symptoms

Therapeutic Nursing Management

- If no previous immunity, rubella vaccine is given to the woman after birth.

- Instruct the client to avoid pregnancy for at least one month if there is exposure to the virus or if post-rubella immunization is provided.

- Controversy in the literature regarding RH immune globulin and rubella vaccine being given to the same woman postpartum. If it is given together postpartum, she should be following up with her health care provider for a blood test to determine if immunity has developed.

Complications

- Rubella acquired in the first trimester is associated with fetal loss and congenital anomalies including intrauterine growth retardation and deafness.

- Intra uterine rubella infection is associated with intrauterine growth retardation.

- Second trimester rubella infection is associated with deafness, congenital cataracts or glaucoma, heart disease, liver impairment with jaundice, chronic pneumonitis, and blood formation disorders, including anemia and thrombocytopenia.

Critical Thinking Exercise: Nursing Management of the Client with Exposure to Rubella

Situation: A.J. has just given birth. She will go home 48 hours after the delivery. She is breastfeeding her baby. Her antepartum rubella titer was 1:8.

1. Should she receive rubella vaccine before leaving the hospital? Why or why not?

2. What questions should the nurse ask A.J. to determine if the rubella vaccine is contraindicated for her? Why?

3. What should the nurse teach A.J. about the vaccine?

Nursing Management of the Client with Placenta Previa

Key Points

- Placenta previa occurs when the placenta implants near or over the cervical os.
- Classic symptom: Painless vaginal bleeding
- Vaginal exams are prohibited in the presence of vaginal bleeding because of the risk of perforating the placenta and causing hemorrhage.
- Nursing care: Monitor for bleeding and onset of labor.
- Medical treatments may include bed rest and intravenous fluids.
- Cesarean birth is usually indicated.
- **Key Terms/Concepts:** Marginal placenta previa, partial placenta previa, total placenta previa, cervical os

Overview

Placenta previa occurs when the placenta implants near or over the cervical os rather than in the uterine fundus. Placenta previa is described as marginal when only an edge of the placenta extends to the internal os; however, it may extend into the os during cervical dilation in labor. Partial placenta previa occurs when the placenta only partially covers the internal os; and total placenta previa means that the internal os is completely covered by the placenta when the cervix is fully dilated. Placenta previa occurs in 1:200 pregnancies. Vaginal exams are prohibited because of the risk for hemorrhage.

Risk Factors

- Uterine scarring (previous uterine surgery)
- Multiple gestation
- History of placenta previa
- Closely-spaced pregnancies
- Uterine tumors
- Increased maternal age
- Endometritis

Signs and Symptoms

- Painless vaginal bleeding (intermittent or in gushes), most commonly occurring in the third trimester
- Progressively more severe bleeding as delivery nears
- Decreasing urinary output

- Anxiety and fear
- Malpresentation or high presenting part

Diagnostic Tests and Lab

- Abdominal ultrasound is done to confirm placental placement and position.
- If hospitalized, perform a non-stress test daily to monitor fetus.

Therapeutic Nursing Management

- Assess amount and character of bleeding.
- Monitor vital signs.
- Monitor urinary output.
- Monitor fetal heart rate and fetal activity continuously.
- Avoid digital vaginal exams.
- Instruct client to avoid enemas, douching, or sexual intercourse.
- Provide bed rest if previa occurs prior to 36 weeks gestation.
- Monitor for continued bleeding and onset of labor.
- Administer intravenous fluid replacement.

Pharmacologic Management

- For preterm labor prior to 34 weeks gestation, administer betamethasone, as prescribed, to promote fetal lung maturity if delivery seems unavoidable.
- Blood transfusion may be needed for severe anemia, chronic abruptio placenta, or placenta previa.

Complications

- Hemorrhage
- Fetal distress/demise related to hypoxia in utero
- Intrauterine growth retardation
- Cesarean delivery
- Preterm birth
- Premature rupture of membranes
- Blood transfusion reactions

Critical Thinking Exercise: Nursing Management of the Client with Placenta Previa

Situation: Elaine, a woman at 33 weeks of gestation is admitted to the hospital with a diagnosis of placenta previa. She is not in labor and is having only mild vaginal bleeding and spotting. Her fetal heart rate is within normal limits for rate and pattern. She is receiving "expectant management" (that is, observation and bed rest) rather than being immediately scheduled for a cesarean birth. Medical orders include the following:

1. Her medical orders appear on the left side of the chart. Write the rationale for these orders and the health teaching that would be included with each one.

Medical Order	Rationale	Teaching
Weekly biophysical profile		
Daily NST		
Weekly CBC		
Physiotherapy consult		
Nutritional consult		
Vital signs q6h (BP, P and FHR)		
Venous access device		
Betamethasone 12 mg IM stat and then repeat in 12 hours		

2. Elaine has a two-year-old at home and a husband who works shift-work. Being on bed rest is a real hardship for her. How would you offer assistance with this?

Nursing Management of the Client with Abruptio Placenta

Key Points

- Abruption is a medical emergency because the risk of maternal hemorrhage and fetal death are significant: 10-30% of clients develop clotting defects (e.g., disseminated intravascular coagulation [DIC]).
- Abruptio placenta should be suspected when there is sudden onset of intense, localized uterine pain, with or without vaginal bleeding.
- Hospitalization is nearly always necessary because the placenta can separate further at any time.
- Vaginal birth is usually feasible.

Overview

Abruptio placenta is the premature separation of only part or of the entire placenta from the uterine wall. Abruption usually occurs in the third trimester. Abruptio placenta occurs in 1% of all deliveries. It is a medical emergency, as approximately 10% of cases of abruption are severe enough to threaten fetal viability. Mild-to-severe abdominal pain and uterine rigidity are usually present and differentiate this condition from placenta previa. Placental abruption requires hospitalization because of the possibility that the placenta can separate further at any time, necessitating immediate delivery. Treatment depends on the severity of blood loss and on fetal maturity and status. Vaginal birth may be feasible, but an emergency cesarean delivery may be indicated in case of fetal distress.

Vaginal bleeding is present in 70-80% of cases, although bleeding may remain concealed (retroplacental hemorrhage). Clinical symptoms vary with degree of separation:

- Grade 1 (mild): Mild vaginal bleeding, mild uterine tenderness; mild uterine tetany; 10-20% of placental surface is detached; neither mother nor fetus is in distress
- Grade 2 (moderate): Uterine tenderness and tetany, with or without external bleeding; mother not in shock, but fetal distress present; about 20-50% of placental surface is detached
- Grade 3 (severe): Severe uterine tetany; woman in shock (although bleeding may not be obvious); fetus is dead; woman often has coagulopathy; more than 50% of placental surface is detached

Risk Factors

- External uterine trauma (blunt trauma)
- Drug abuse during pregnancy, especially cocaine
- Pregnancy-induced hypertension
- Previous abruption
- Folic acid deficiency
- Smoking
- Cocaine use
- Premature rupture of membranes
- Maternal hypertension: this is the most consistently identified risk factor
- Multifetal pregnancies
- Short umbilical cord

Diagnostic Tests and Lab

- Hemoglobin
- Hematocrit
- Ultrasound of abdomen
- Blood type and crossmatch
- Coagulation profile
- Sonogram (to rule out placenta previa)

Signs and Symptoms

- Dark red vaginal bleeding
- Uterine rigidity
- Sudden onset of intense abdominal pain
- Uterine contractions
- Fetal distress

Therapeutic Nursing Management

- Assess amount and character of bleeding.
- Assess degree of abdominal rigidity.
- Assess degree of abdominal pain.
- Assess fetal activity and heart tones.
- Measure fundal height if concealed bleeding is suspected.
- Monitor for shock (vital signs, urine output, physical assessment).
- Provide emotional support because the family may be experiencing fetal loss in addition to a critical illness.
- Prepare woman for possible emergency cesarean delivery.
- Administer blood transfusions if ordered.

Complications

- Severely compromised fetal well-being
- Fetal demise (frequent if separation is 50% or greater)
- Maternal disseminated intravascular coagulopathy (DIC)
- Concealed central placental bleed
- Shock

Critical Thinking Exercise: Nursing Management of the Client with Abruptio Placenta

Situation: A woman at 35 weeks of gestation is admitted to the hospital with a small amount of vaginal bleeding and moderately severe abdominal pain. The fetal heart rate is within normal limits for rate and pattern. Her blood pressure has been elevated for the past month, and is 160/90 today. Her pulse is 80, temperature is 98.6° F, and respirations are 14. The nursing history reveals that she is underweight and does not maintain a healthy diet. She says, "I don't know how I can stand to stay here if you don't let me smoke." Medical orders include the following:

- Continuous electronic fetal monitoring
- Indwelling urinary catheter
- Intravenous fluids
- Give betamethasone (a glucocorticoid) 12 mg intramuscular q12hrs x two doses

1. What are the risk factors that may have contributed to this woman's placental abruption?

2. Why was an indwelling urinary catheter ordered?

3. Why were intravenous fluids ordered?

4. While you are assisting her to her birthing room, reviewing her obstetrical history and vital signs, you observe her increasing distress with pain. Your abdominal palpation suggests that her abdomen is becoming more taut and tender. The fetal heart rate baseline has decreased from 120 bpm to 108 bpm. What is your plan of care for this woman/family?

5. How would you describe your plan of care to this woman/family?

6. What is the most logical explanation for what is happening?

Nursing Management of the Client with Exposure to Infections

Key Points

- Toxoplasmosis
- Other (gonorrhea, syphilis, varicella, hepatitis B, group B streptococci, and human immunodeficiency virus)
- Rubella
- Cytomegalovirus (CMV)
- Herpes
- All **TORCH** infections can cross the placenta.
- Prenatal screening is important because although many infections are asymptomatic or produce vague, influenza-like symptoms, they can cause serious fetal and neonatal effects.
- Prenatal complications include premature labor and premature rupture of membranes.
- Neonatal complications include congenital heart (and other) defects, mental retardation, and encephalitis.
- Streptococcus (Group B) is a frequent cause of preterm labor, as well as sepsis in the mother and neonate.
- **Key Terms/Concepts:** TORCH, STDs, GBS, preterm labor and delivery

Overview

TORCH infections during pregnancy place the woman and fetus in jeopardy due to the associated complications. TORCH stands for T toxoplasmosis, O other, R rubella, C cytomegalovirus (CMV), H herpes ("other" includes gonorrhea, syphilis, varicella, hepatitis B, group B streptococci, and human immunodeficiency virus). TORCH-related complications include: congenital heart defects, physical fetal anomalies, intrauterine growth retardation (IUGR), mental retardation, and encephalitis, hydrocephalus, or porencephaly.

Risk Factors

- Pregnancy-related or physiologic (e.g., urinary tract infections)
- Exposure to teratogenic infections
- Sexually transmitted disease (gonorrhea, syphilis, chlamydia, herpes, HIV/AIDS, hepatitis B, TB)
- Children at day care centers have a high risk of acquiring CMV.
- Toxoplasmosis parasite found in cat litter

Diagnostic Tests and Lab

- Screening for infections throughout pregnancy (TORCH titer, IgM, or IgG)
- Diagnostic tests depend on the type of infection (e.g., toxoplasmosis and rubella titers).

Signs and Symptoms

Although some maternal symptoms are disease specific, many TORCH infections are asymptomatic or produce vague, nonspecific symptoms. For example, cytomegalovirus (CMV) acquired in adulthood may resemble the common cold. Therefore, serologic screening is important throughout pregnancy.

Examples of some symptoms are as follow:

- Fatigue
- Enlarged lymph nodes
- Fever
- Mono-like symptoms
- Genital infection
- Cervical inflammation
- Rash

Therapeutic Nursing Management

- Treat for specific infection per primary care provider's orders.
- Implement universal precautions by all health care providers.
- Administer hepatitis B immune globulin (HBIG) to the infant within the first 12 hours after birth if the maternal status is positive for the screening antigen (HBsAg) or the status is unknown.
- Administer hepatitis B vaccine (HBV) to the infant within the first 12 hours after birth if the maternal status is positive for the screening antigen (HBsAg) or the status is unknown.
- Monitor fetal status.
- Take frequent vital signs.

Complications

Some infections produce complications prenatally (e.g., premature labor, premature rupture of membranes). All TORCH infections may infect the fetus/neonate, producing neonatal complications.

Gonorrhea caused by *neisseria gonorrhea*, can be transmitted to the neonate during birth. C-section is advised to avoid transmission. Mother is treated with antibiotics. The related fetal complications include spontaneous abortion, preterm delivery, and premature rupture of membranes (PROM). Neonatal risks include gonococcal ophthalmia, which can cause blindness. Erythromycin (Ilotycin) ointment is administered at birth to prevent ophthalmia neonatorum.

Congenital syphilis is caused by maternal transmission either in utero or at delivery. If the mother is treated successfully with penicillin before the 18th week of pregnancy, the neonate will not likely develop syphilis. Related complications include spontaneous abortion, neonatal infection, fetal death, stillbirth, and preterm delivery. Disorders of the central nervous system (CNS), teeth, and cornea may become evident several months after birth.

Chlamydia causes premature rupture of membranes, preterm labor and early delivery, low birth weight, conjunctivitis, pneumonia, opthalmia neonatorum, and chronic otitis media. Although it is usually asymptomatic in the mother, it can cause bleeding, purulent vaginal discharge, pelvic inflammatory disease, or dysuria. It is treated with erythromycin or amoxicillin.

Herpes is caused by the herpes simplex virus (HSV), and is spread during the birth process if the woman has active lesions, usually with primary infection. The neonate is highly contagious and should be isolated. Antiviral drugs are given to the neonate, but they are not approved for use in pregnancy. Herpes infection during pregnancy can cause spontaneous abortion, preterm labor, and intrauterine growth retardation. In the neonate, HSV causes local neonatal infection (skin, eyes, nose); systemic infections of the liver, CNS, or other organs; seizures; jaundice; and skin lesions.

Fetal/Newborn HIV/AIDS destroys the body's immune system and there is no cure.

Hepatitis B causes newborn symptoms of fever, jaundice, and enlarged liver. The complication of pregnancy is preterm labor.

CMV (cytomegalovirus) is a perinatal infection, often asymptomatic or present with flu-like symptoms in the mother. One-quarter to one-third of all women have had CMV infection at some time (evidenced by positive serologic markers), although it is the primary infection during pregnancy that can cause neonatal disease. Congenital infection may result in newborn mental retardation, congenital deafness, hydrocephalus, microcephaly, mental retardation, hearing loss, or learning disabilities. Death occurs shortly after birth. Blood transfusions are now screened for CMV and avoided for use during pregnancy and during the newborn period. There is no effective prevention or treatment.

Toxoplasmosis is a protozoan. The mother acquires the pathogen from poorly cooked meat or cat feces, and it is transferred to the fetus through the placenta. Maternal symptoms include malaise, lymphadenopathy, muscle pain, and slight fever. Spontaneous abortion may result. Fetal/newborn symptoms include hydrocephalus, blindness, deafness, or mental retardation. Perinatal damage is not reversible. Drug therapy is pyrimethamine or sulfadiazine.

Rubella is caused by the rubella virus. When the mother is exposed during pregnancy, the fetus acquires the infection in utero. Prevention is achieved by rubella vaccination. There is no treatment. In the neonate, rubella can cause congenital cataracts, congenital heart disease, deafness, intrauterine growth retardation, and extremity malformation.

Streptococcus (Group B) may be acquired throughout pregnancy and childbirth, and is treated with antibiotics. Women can carry the bacterium but not have symptoms. Fetal/ newborn complications include preterm labor, premature rupture of membranes, chorioamnionitis, stillbirth, respiratory distress syndrome, apnea, and shock. It may cause urinary tract infections in the mother, as well as postpartum sepsis.

Thrush caused by candida albicans (yeast) is a vaginal infection in the mother, is highly contagious, and is transmitted to the newborn at birth. It is treated with Mycostatin. Oral candidiasis produces small white patches on the newborn's buccal membranes and tongue.

Critical Thinking Exercise: Nursing Management of the Client with Exposure to Infections

Situation: At her first prenatal visit, a woman says, "My friend had TORCH infection when she was pregnant, and her baby died. Can I get an immunization to prevent that disease?"

1. How should the nurse answer this question?

2. The woman says, "What can I do to keep from getting these infections and passing them to my baby?" What advice should the nurse give to her?

3. For which of the TORCH infections are immunizations available?

Nursing Management of the Client with Substance Use

Key Points

- Any use of alcohol or street or recreational drugs during pregnancy is considered substance use.
- Tobacco and alcohol are the most frequently used substances in pregnancy.
- Prenatal alcohol exposure is the most common preventable cause of mental retardation.
- Risk factors for substance use include psychiatric illness, physical or sexual abuse, and low self-esteem.
- **Key Terms/Concepts:** Alcohol, illicit drugs, tobacco, neonatal abstinence syndrome

Overview

Substance use is addiction to, or continued use of, an illegal or prescribed substance/drug even though it is causing physical, social, or interpersonal problems. Any use of alcohol or illicit drugs during pregnancy is considered "abuse" because of the serious effects on the fetus and neonate. Such substances include nicotine, alcohol, cocaine, marijuana, narcotics, hallucinogens, stimulants, sleeping pills, tranquilizers, and pain relievers. Maternal substance use during the first trimester places the fetus at the greatest risk. Risk increases with the strength, amount, frequency, and route of administration. In addition to fetal risk, drug use can disturb relationships, create dependency, and cause serious health problems. Alcohol use during pregnancy is the leading cause of mental retardation in the United States. Every pregnant woman should be screened for substance use (at least verbally) at the first prenatal visit, so that intervention can begin early. However, women who use drugs often do not receive prenatal care.

Risk Factors

- Age (e.g., women ages 21-34 have the highest rates of specific alcohol-related problems during pregnancy)
- Previous alcohol and tobacco use
- Sexual promiscuity
- Depression and anxiety disorders
- Low self-esteem
- Insomnia
- Physical or sexual abuse

Diagnostic Tests and Lab

- Urine toxicology screen
- Serum toxicology screen

Signs and Symptoms

Specific signs and symptoms depend on the substance being used/abused.

- Signs of **maternal addiction** to some kind of drug include
  - Constricted pupils
  - Dental caries
  - Mood swings
  - Rhinitis
  - Frequent falls/accidents
  - Anorexia
  - Weight loss
  - Poor hygiene
  - No prenatal care
  - Irregular, fast heart rate
  - Recurrence of sexually transmitted diseases
- Signs of **withdrawal in newborn** hours after birth
  - Listlessness
  - Poor muscle reflexes
  - Poor feeding; uncoordinated suck, swallow
  - High-pitched cry
  - Jitteriness/tremors
  - Restless sleeping
  - Inability to be consoled when crying

Therapeutic Nursing Management

- Identify drug use early; incorporate questions or self-report questionnaires into routine prenatal interviews.
- Intervene and encourage client to decrease drug use and join support program to facilitate withdrawal and improve general health.
- Refer for rehabilitation.
- Be aware of laws regarding prenatal drug use. In some states, the child must be referred to child protective services.

Maternal Complications

- High blood pressure
- Anemia
- Nutritional deficiencies
- Pancreatitis
- Alcoholic hepatitis and cirrhosis

Complications in Fetus and Newborn

- Newborn addiction and withdrawal
- Abruptio placenta
- Fetus: Intrauterine growth retardation (cocaine, heroin, amphetamines)
- Fetal alcohol syndrome (FAS)—Prenatal and postnatal growth restriction; central nervous system malfunctions (including mental retardation); and facial features such as microcephaly, small eyes, flattened nasal bridge, and a thin upper lip. FAS may also include other craniofacial anomalies. The incidence of learning delays and behavioral abnormalities, such as attention deficit hyperactivity disorder (ADHD) or oppositional behavioral disorder, are greater in children exposed to alcohol prenatally.
- Long-term learning disabilities and delayed language development
- Tobacco effects: Prematurity, low birth weight; increased risk for respiratory disorders, developmental delays, and sudden infant death syndrome

Critical Thinking Exercise: Nursing Management of the Client with Substance Use

Situation: An adolescent comes to the clinic for the first time when she is in the third trimester of pregnancy. She has gained only five pounds over her stated prepregnant weight. Her partner states that they have an occasional beer on the weekend.

1. How should the nurse proceed to assess this client for substance abuse?

2. The client admits to smoking and "drinking quite a bit of coffee" and other caffeinated beverages. She finally tells the nurse that she drinks beer, "at least one or two a day," and that she sometimes takes "speed" to wake up when she is "hung over" from drinking. Because the client is clearly using substances, what other conditions should the nurse suspect and screen for?

3. Why was verbal screening necessary? What does the nurse need to do to obtain a urine- screening test for substances?

Nursing Management of the Pregnant Adolescent

Key Points

- Adolescents are less likely to seek early prenatal care.
- Adolescents are more likely to smoke and less likely to gain adequate weight.
- The younger the adolescent, the higher the risk of poor pregnancy outcomes.
- Goals of nursing are to (1) encourage early and continued prenatal care and (2) refer the adolescent for social and economic support, as needed.
- The birth rate for adolescents has declined steadily since 1991; however, the U.S. still has the highest adolescent birth rate among industrialized countries.
- **Key Terms/Concepts**: Adolescence, impulsivity

Overview

The United States has the highest incidence of adolescent pregnancy among western countries. Most teenage pregnancies are unplanned. Adolescents are less likely to seek early prenatal care and are more likely to be noncompliant in the areas of nutrition and prenatal care. When prenatal care is lacking, there is higher risk for pregnancy-induced hypertension, preterm birth, and intrauterine growth restriction. Prenatal care does improve outcomes. Psychosocial risks include high divorce rates, single-parent families, disrupted education, and low income.

In a teenager 16 years of age or younger, pregnancy introduces additional physical and emotional stress on an already stressful developmental period. Teenagers are commonly impulsive and self-centered, and do not plan for the future. This places their children at risk for abuse and neglect, partly because of teens' inadequate knowledge.

Risk Factors—Factors Contributing to Teenage Pregnancy

- Cohabitation
- Premarital sex
- Poverty
- Low self-esteem
- Ethnic considerations–highest in African American, Hispanic, and Native American teens
- Households with a single parent
- Risk-taking behaviors
- History of alcohol and drug abuse
- Juvenile delinquency

Therapeutic Nursing Management

- Assess nutritional status and teach about good nutrition.
- Assess knowledge base and instruct about labor, delivery, and postpartum expectations.
- Provide education regarding newborn care.
- Provide resources such as clothing, money, and food.
- Teach how pregnancy occurred and about use of birth control after delivery.
- Teach pregnancy prevention and infection measures.
- Obtain baseline weight and blood pressure.
- Obtain immunization history.
- Assess support systems.
- Explore attitudes and feelings regarding the pregnancy and the newborn.
- Assess bonding after delivery.
- Promote healthy infant stimulation activities.
- Seek community resources, such as *Parents as Teachers*, to provide follow-up assessment and education to the mother.

Complications

- Financial strain, due to expense of clothing, feeding, and sheltering mother and baby, as well as added child care costs or altered employment.
- Maternal educational goals postponed
- Infant abuse or abandonment related to poor parenting skills
- Pregnancy-induced hypertension
- Infection
- Anemia
- Infant failure to thrive

Critical Thinking Exercise: Nursing Management of the Pregnant Adolescent

Situation: B.K., a 15-year-old adolescent in her sixth month of pregnancy, has come to the clinic for her first prenatal visit. She lives at home with her parents, and will continue to do so after the birth of the baby. B.K. says she does not know who the baby's father is.

1. Because of B.K.'s age, what assessments are especially important to make?

2. Why is the transition to parenthood especially difficult for adolescent parents?

3. For what physical complications are B.K. and her baby at especially high risk?

4. In order to promote a healthy pregnancy, what is the most important nursing intervention at this time?

Nursing Management of the Client Requiring an Amniocentesis

Key Points

- Amniocentesis is an invasive procedure that requires (1) a signed consent form and (2) sterile technique.
- Ultrasonography is used to direct the procedure.
- Amniocentesis is performed to evaluate fetal status (e.g., maturity, congenital anomalies).
- Complications, although not common, include maternal and fetal hemorrhage, infection, injury from the needle, and preterm labor.
- Nursing responsibilities include teaching the client about the procedure, maintaining sterile technique, monitoring for complications, and teaching the client about self-care afterward.

Overview

Amniocentesis involves the withdrawal of a sample of amniotic fluid, which contains fetal cells, for laboratory analysis. Indicated to measure fetal maturity and to rule out congenital abnormalities, genetic defects, or intrauterine growth retardation, amniotic fluid sampling is usually performed after 14 weeks gestation. Direct ultrasonographic visualization is used and a needle is inserted transabdominally into the uterus. Amniotic fluid is then drawn into a syringe. Complications occur in less than 1% of cases.

Diagnostic Tests and Labs

AFP: Alpha-fetoprotein is an antigen carried by the fetus. Elevated levels indicate neural tube defects. Low levels may indicate Down's syndrome.

Ultrasonography: Determines fetal/placental position.

Creatinine level: Level of less than 1.8 mg/dL demonstrates maturing kidney function of fetus.

L/S (lecithin/sphingomyelin ratio): Ratio of 2:1 indicates fetal lung maturity.

Phosphatidylglycerol (PG): When present with a 2:1 L/S ratio, helps confirm fetal maturity.

Shake test: Amniotic fluid is mixed with saline and ethanol and vigorously shaken. Appearance of bubbles that float and remain for 15 minutes indicates fetal lung maturity.

Bilirubin level: Indicates degree of destruction of fetal red blood cells in an Rh-sensitized woman.

Therapeutic Nursing Management

- Assist with procedure, monitor for sterility.
- Determine whether the client is to empty her bladder before the procedure. A full bladder enhances the ultrasound imaging; an empty bladder reduces the risk of perforating the bladder with the amniocentesis needle.
- Position client in left lateral tilt to prevent hypotension during the procedure.
- Provide emotional support.
- Refer client for genetic counseling when indicated.
- Women who are Rh negative receive Rh0 (D) immune globulin (RhoGAM) after the procedure because of the possibility of maternal Rh isoimmunization.
- This procedure usually requires signing an informed consent form, including a clear explanation of risks of the procedure.
- Use universal precautions, including eye goggles, during the procedure.

Complications

- Needle puncture of the fetus
- Bleeding caused by perforation of placenta
- Loss of amniotic fluid
- Infection
- Premature labor
- Spontaneous abortion
- Fetal distress

Critical Thinking Exercise: Nursing Management of the Client Requiring an Amniocentesis

Situation: L.L. is 20 weeks pregnant. She has signed a consent form and is having an amniocentesis so that amniotic fluid can be obtained. Her maternal serum screening test came back with a high chance of spina bifida. She has determined with her partner and genetic counselor that she would like to rule out any false positives or negatives and to know for sure if her baby will have spina bifida. After the initial ultrasonography, the nurse directs L.L. to empty her bladder before the amniocentesis is performed.

1. Why was it necessary for L.L. to empty her bladder?

2. Why was ultrasonography used along with amniocentesis?

3. The obstetrician states that he needs to inform L.L. of the risks and benefits of this procedure. What will be included in his discussion with L.L.?

4. What assessments should be made after the procedure?

Nursing Management of the Client Requiring Contraction Stress and Non-Stress Test Monitoring

Key Points

- NST and CST use the fetal heart rate and pattern to assess fetal well-being.
- Non-stress test (NST):
    - Evaluates FHR in response to fetal movement
    - Reactive (normal)=2-4 FHR accelerations in 10 minutes
    - No side effects
- Contraction stress test (CST):
    - Evaluates FHR in response to uterine contractions
    - Negative (normal)=no late FHR decelerations produced by uterine contractions
    - Possible side effects: overstimulation of the uterus secondary to use of oxytocin
- **Key Terms/Concepts**: NST, CST, non-reassuring, reassuring, negative, positive, client teaching, accelerations, late decelerations

Overview

Electronic fetal monitoring is used to assess fetal well-being during the antepartal period and during labor and delivery. In the first and second trimesters, it is intended mainly for diagnosis of fetal anomalies; in the third trimester it is used to determine whether the intrauterine environment is still supportive of the fetus that is, whether to induce delivery or allow the pregnancy to continue. As a rule, a reactive non-stress test and a negative contraction stress test are associated with favorable birth outcomes.

The non-stress test (NST) is the most widely used antepartum test of fetal status. It is noninvasive, relatively inexpensive, and there are no side effects or contraindications. It is based on the theory that a normal fetus will produce characteristic heart rate patterns in response to its body movements (e.g., heart rate will increase with movement). A reactive test (FHR accelerations with fetal movement) provides reassurance of fetal well-being. However, a non-reactivity does not necessarily indicate a problem. Non-reactivity may be caused by fetal sleep, medications, and fetal immaturity. A nonreactive test usually requires further assessments (e.g., with a CST or biophysical profile)

The contraction stress test (CST) assesses the fetal heart rate (FHR) response to uterine contractions. The purpose is to assess fetal ability to tolerate the stress of labor. In a healthy fetus, contractions should not produce hypoxia and FHR changes. However, if there is underlying uteroplacental insufficiency, contractions will produce late decelerations in the FHR. If the woman is not having spontaneous contractions, the uterus is stimulated by means of manual nipple stimulation or intravenous oxytocin administration. CST is an invasive procedure and because the uterus can be overstimulated, the CST is contraindicated in some conditions (e.g., placenta previa, multifetal pregnancy, incompetent cervix, rupture of membranes).

Risk Factors—Indications for NST/CST

- Pregnancy-induced hypertension
- Diabetes
- Placenta previa
- Abruptio placenta
- Post maturity
- Decreased fetal activity

Diagnostic Tests and Labs

- NST is considered reactive (normal) when there are 2-4 FHR accelerations in 10 minutes. Accelerations are an increase in FHR by 10-15 beats and lasting 15 seconds. High rate of false-nonreactive results occurs because of fetal sleep cycles, medications, and fetal immaturity.
- CST is considered negative (normal) when the woman is having three contractions in a 10-minute period, and no late FHR decelerations are produced by the contractions.

Therapeutic Nursing Management

- Position woman on left side or in semi-Fowlers.
- Apply conduction gel and secure external ultrasound transducer to abdomen. Apply tocodynamometer to fundus to assess contractions/fetal movement.
- Monitor the maternal and fetal response to the test.
- Increase intravenous oxytocin dosage every 15 minutes until three contractions are obtained. Monitor fetal heart rate and uterine contractions electronically (for CST).
- When there is no fetal movement during a NST, the nurse can attempt to stimulate fetal activity by using a transvaginal light, manipulating the woman's abdomen, or having her drink orange juice; however, research has not shown any of these to be very effective.
- For NST, vibroacoustic stimulation has been shown to be somewhat effective in stimulating fetal movement.

Complications

- CST may cause fetal distress (fetal distress is indicated by **decelerations**— decrease in FHR after contraction begins and failure to return to prior rate until after the contraction ends).
- CST may cause labor.
- CST may cause hyperstimulation of the uterus if oxytocin is used.
- NST has no associated complications.

Critical Thinking Exercise: Nursing Management of the Client Requiring Contraction Stress and Non-Stress Test Monitoring

Situation: A woman at 33 weeks of gestation is having a non-stress test. The nurse seats her comfortably in a reclining chair and places a Doppler transducer and a Tocotransducer on her abdomen. She hands the woman a hand-held device with a button on the end.

1. The woman asks, "What am I supposed to do with this button thing?" What instructions should the nurse give her?

2. The woman asks, "Will this take very long? I have to meet a client at 3 o'clock." What should the nurse tell her?

3. After 20 minutes, no fetal movements have occurred and no FHR accelerations have been noted. The woman says, "Are we all through now?" What should the nurse tell her?

4. The woman says, "My sister had a stress test and it put her into labor. I'm not even near my due date. Will that happen to me?" What should the nurse tell her?

5. After 10 more minutes, the monitor shows three FHR accelerations of 12 beats per minute, lasting 20 seconds each. Is this a reactive or a nonreactive test? Is that a reassuring finding, or not?

Case Study: The Antepartum Client

Situation: A 23-year-old client and her husband are expecting their first baby. The client thinks she is about 10 weeks pregnant, and this is her first prenatal visit. She and her husband speak fluent Spanish, but have difficulty speaking English. They have many questions and are excited about the baby. All laboratory tests and the physical exam are within normal limits. The nurse plans to begin some antepartum teaching during this clinic visit.

Instructions: With a partner, list the danger signs of pregnancy that you will teach the client and her husband. Identify two ways you can teach the information.

DANGER SIGNS	TEACHING METHODS

The client returns for her 16-week checkup to the clinic. Her vital signs are 118/80, pulse 80, respirations 16. Her urine studies are normal, but her hemoglobin is 11.0 gm/dL and hematocrit is 32%.

Which foods should the nurse advise the client to eat?

At the next clinic visit, the client is scheduled to have a routine ultrasound of her fetus. What will you do to prepare her for the event?

Instructions: Write a paragraph or two detailing the instructions and information you would give the client about the ultrasonography.

Interactive Activity: How do you teach material containing the danger signs of pregnancy without alarming the client? How do you know they are learned? What kinds of written materials or audiovisuals might be helpful?

Nursing Management of the Client Preparing for Labor

> ## Key Points
>
> - The intrapartum nurse actually has three clients that require constant monitoring: the mother, the fetus, and the family unit.
> - Factors affecting labor and birth (the 5 Ps): passenger, passageway, powers, position, and psychological response.
> - The uterine contraction pattern, dilation and effacement of the cervix, and the descent of the fetus determine labor progression.
> - Stages of labor:
>   - First stage, latent: Cervical dilation 0-3 cm. This is the longest phase.
>   - First stage, active: Cervical dilation 4-8 cm
>   - First stage, transition: Cervical dilation 8-10 cm (full dilation)
>   - Second stage (stage of expulsion): From full cervical dilation through birth of the baby
>   - Third stage: From birth of the baby through expulsion of the placenta (5-30 minutes)
>   - Fourth stage: The first four hours after delivery
> - **Key Terms/Concepts:** Premonitory signs of labor, true labor/false labor, dystocia, cervical dilation, cervical effacement, contractions, rupture of membranes, fetal station (descent)

Overview

Labor is the series of processes by which the fetus is expelled from the uterus. The mother and fetus undergo physiologic adaptations during pregnancy: the mother, to prepare for birth; and the fetus, to prepare for extrauterine life. Several weeks before actual labor begins, the client may experience physical changes that alert her to the approach of labor. It is important for the nurse to recognize and teach the client the difference between true and false labor.

Factors that Affect the Process of Labor and Birth

It may help to remember these factors as "the 5 Ps": passenger, passageway, powers, position, and psychologic response. Conditions that cause any of these to be ineffective (e.g., maternal fatigue, shoulder presentation of the fetus) can impede labor. For example, the uterine and abdominal muscles of a multiparous woman may not be strong enough to move the fetus effectively.

Passenger (fetus and placenta): Fetal presentation, position, attitude, and lie. Station and engagement are assessments of fetal position.

Passageway (birth canal, bony pelvis, cervix, vagina): Size and shape of the bony pelvis must allow room for passage of fetus. Prenatal pelvic measurements provide this information. Cervix must dilate and efface sufficiently to allow fetus to descend into the vagina.

Powers (involuntary uterine contractions and voluntary, "bearing-down" efforts to expel the fetus): Strong, effective contractions are needed. Involuntary contractions are responsible for dilating and effacing the cervix and causing fetal descent. After full cervical dilation, voluntary bearing-down is needed to expel the infant from the uterus and vagina.

Position (maternal): The actual position the mother assumes for labor and birth. For pushing, this is usually a semirecumbent position.

Psychological response: Labor and birth are both exciting and anxiety-producing. Maternal stress and tension can produce physiologic responses that interfere with labor and stress the fetus.

Signs and Symptoms

Premonitory signs: Signs and symptoms of impending labor.

Lightening: 14 days before labor, primigravidas may notice the baby has moved into the pelvis or "dropped." Women experience relief of pressure on the diaphragm and increased pressure on the bladder. Multiparas do not experience "lightening."

Cervical changes: Softening and hyperplasia signal labor. These changes must be detected by vaginal exam. Dilation and effacement signal labor progression.

Weight loss: Clients experience a 1-3 pound weight loss before labor begins. Gastrointestinal disturbances may also be present, such as nausea, indigestion, or constipation.

Backache: low, dull backache and mild cramping are characteristic of the onset of labor.

Energy burst: 24-48 hours prior to labor onset, a client may experience a burst of energy, otherwise known as "nesting."

Contractions: They progress from the top of the uterus and spread throughout the uterus. Contractions should increase in frequency and intensity as labor progresses. The frequency of contractions is determined by measuring the length of time from the beginning of one contraction to the beginning of the next contraction.

Ruptured membranes: Most women go into labor within 24 hours after membranes have ruptured. Prolonged rupture of membranes before delivery of the fetus may lead to infection.

True versus False Labor

Key: True labor produces cervical dilation and effacement.

TRUE LABOR	FALSE LABOR
Contractions	Contractions
Regular	Irregular or regular for short periods
Becoming stronger, longer, closer together	Stop with walking or position changes
Felt in lower back, radiate to abdomen	Felt above navel
Not stopped with comfort measures or hydration	Can be stopped by use of comfort measures or hydration

TRUE LABOR	FALSE LABOR
Cervix (vaginal exam) Progressive change (dilation, effacement) Bloody show present Increasingly anterior position	**Cervix (vaginal exam)** No change (may be soft) Often posterior No bloody show
Fetus Usually engaged in pelvis	**Fetus** Usually not engaged

Stages of Labor

First stage: The stage of cervical effacement and dilation. The cervix dilates fully, to 10 cm, by the end of the first stage. Consists of latent, active, and transition phases:

- **Latent phase:** The cervix dilates from 0-4 cm. Early in this phase, the contractions may be irregular, 10-20 minutes apart, and lasting 15-30 seconds. Clients experience cramping, low backache and bloody show. Administering analgesics during this phase of labor may space out the contractions and prolong labor. Latent phase averages 8-20 hours for primigravidas; 5-14 hours for multiparas.

- **Active phase:** Begins when the cervix is dilated to 3 cm and lasts to 7 or 8 cm. Contractions are 3-5 minutes apart, of moderate intensity, and last 30-60 seconds. Clients experience growing discomfort. Membranes may rupture.

- **Transition phase:** 8-10 cm to full dilation. Contractions occur every 2-3 minutes, are intense, and are 60-90 seconds in duration. Bloody show increases. Clients experience extreme discomfort and may have a strong desire to push in this phase, even though not fully dilated.

Second stage: The stage of expulsion. The second stage begins with full cervical dilation and ends at the birth of the neonate. Contractions are very intense, every 1-2 minutes, and last 60-90 seconds. Involuntary contractions and maternal pushing accomplish expulsion of the fetus.

Third stage: The stage of placental expulsion. The third stage ends at the delivery of the placenta. Average duration of this stage is 5-30 minutes. Detachment of the placenta is indicated by the lengthening of the umbilical cord.

Fourth stage: The stage of recovery. The fourth stage encompasses the first four hours after delivery. The client's physiologic stability is restored. Bonding activities are important in this stage.

Therapeutic Nursing Management (True vs. False Labor)

- Advise client to change her activity level to differentiate false labor from true. Walking is the activity of choice. True labor will usually intensify with increased client activity; false labor may stop.

- Provide adequate hydration to avoid "false labor" (dehydrated clients may cease contractions following intravenous hydration).

- Reassure clients who are embarrassed about being admitted to the hospital in "false labor" that it is difficult to tell the difference and that many women, even nurses, can misinterpret the signs of labor.

Therapeutic Nursing Management (Stages of Labor)

- During first stage (latent phase), nurses may orient the client and family to labor and delivery as they monitor labor progress. Frequent position changes can help the fetus rotate and descend into the birth canal.

- As active labor begins, pain control and client/fetal monitoring are important.

- In transition, the nurse comforts the client and prepares for second stage. The client should be discouraged from pushing until she is fully dilated to help reduce the risk of cervical lacerations.

- In second stage, the nurse assists in pushing as appropriate and prepares for the birth of the baby and the placenta.

- In fourth stage, the nurse monitors vital signs, fundal height and firmness, lochia, urinary output, and bonding activities.

Complications of Labor

- Infection
- Cord compression
- Cephalopelvic disproportion
- Dystocia
- Failure to progress
- Breech presentation/shoulder presentation
- Fetal anomalies
- Preterm labor and birth
- Post-term dates
- Meconium passage prior to delivery can result in meconium aspiration syndrome.
- Hemorrhage
- Tugging on or twisting the umbilical cord puts client at risk for hemorrhage or retained placenta.
- Fourth stage labor involves risk of hemorrhage, hypotension, urinary retention, and reaction to medications or anesthesia.

Critical Thinking Exercise: Nursing Management of the Client Preparing for Labor

Situation: A 24-year-old woman, gravida 1, TPAL 0000 at 40 weeks gestation, has come to the birth setting because she thinks she is in labor. She tells you that she felt the baby "drop" over the last two weeks and that she has been having contractions for the past two hours. She reports that she has not had any fluid leaking from her vagina and that she does not think her membranes have ruptured. She says, "My contractions are coming every 15 minutes and they last for about 30 seconds. They don't change when I lie down or walk about. I think I saw some bloody show, but I'm not sure. Do you think my labor has started?"

1. What signs of true labor does this woman have?

2. How can the nurse determine whether or not this is true labor?

3. How should the nurse answer the woman's question about whether or not she is in labor?

4. The nurse does an abdominal assessment of the woman's contractions and determines that they are moderate in strength. The woman's vital signs are within normal limits and the fetal heart rate is 136 bpm (measured for one full minute following a contraction). She also performs a digital examination of the client's cervix and finds that it is dilated to 2 cm and 50% effaced. She checks again in an hour and finds that the cervical dilation is between 2 and 3 cm and that the cervix is now about 80% effaced. The uterine contraction pattern remains the same, except that the contractions are now 45-50 seconds in duration. The nurse performs a Nitrazine paper test and confirms that the woman's membranes are intact. What stage and phase of labor do these findings indicate?

5. Vandevusse has described additional P's or essential forces of labor. A few have been listed in this table. Describe the effect they may have on labor and what the nurse could do to assist the woman/family.

Additional P's	Effect	Nursing Assessment/ Interventions
Preparations by Mother, e.g., Prenatal Class attendance		
Professional providers, e.g. Presence of the nurse in labor		
Procedures, e.g. Requiring a woman to wear a hospital gown in labor		

Nursing Management of the Client with Pain: Nonpharmacologic

Key Points

- Pain experience and pain tolerance vary widely among individuals.
- Nonpharmacologic pain control measures seek to reduce fear and tension, major causes of pain in labor.
- Measures such as effleurage and counterpressure make use of the gate-control theory to relieve pain.
- Nonpharmacologic measures include acupressure, heat and cold applications, therapeutic touch, hypnosis, biofeedback, aromatherapy, music, use of a TENS unit, water therapy, and breathing techniques.
- Common childbirth preparation methods are Dick-Read, Lamaze, and Bradley.
- Frequent position changes promote relaxation.
- **Key Terms/Concepts:** Effleurage, gate-control therapy, Lamaze, breathing techniques, client teaching

Overview

Nonpharmacologic comfort measures are those that reduce pain without use of analgesics or anesthesia. Many variables influence pain during childbirth, for example: physical (fatigue, fetal size and position), psychological (response to pain, fear), sociocultural (pain perception and cultural expectations for pain behaviors), and environmental (noise and activity levels). The fear-tension-pain syndrome is a series of client responses to pain: as pain increases, so do fear and anxiety, which become a vicious cycle because an anxious client has heightened perception of painful stimuli. Fear-tension-pain may cause the client to hyperventilate, to cry out, writhe, scream, and/ or be unable to follow instructions. Tolerance for and expressions of pain vary widely among individuals. Some nonpharmacologic measures (acupressure, hypnosis, and therapeutic touch) require special training.

Risk Factors

- Fear
- Anxiety
- Fatigue
- Pain cycle
- Uterine/birth canal stretching in labor
- Individual pain tolerance variations
- Malposition of the fetus
- Cephalopelvic disproportion (CPD)

Signs and Symptoms of Pain

- Increased blood pressure
- Tachycardia
- Behavioral manifestations
- Fatigue
- Crying, screaming
- Hyperventilation
- Moaning
- Inability to follow instructions
- Writhing
- Withdrawal or avoidance behaviors

Causes of Labor Pain

First stage labor pain is a result of uterine contractions, stretching of the uterus, and dilating and effacing of the cervical os. Fetal presentation may add to the discomfort, such as in a posterior presentation. Discomfort is typically in the back and radiates to the abdomen.

Second stage labor pain results in pain and extreme pressure on the perineum and the muscles of the vagina as the fetus pushes forward. Second stage uterine contractions increase in intensity, frequency, and duration.

Third stage labor pain occurs as uterine contractions expel the placenta.

Therapeutic Nursing Management

- Provide information to assist the client in reducing pain.
- Assist client to shower to reduce pain and foster comfort.
- Physical touch is soothing in early labor. Try back rubs, back support, and effleurage.
- Apply cool cloth to forehead between contractions.
- Use warmed blankets or a moist heating pad to relieve muscle ischemia and increase blood flow to the area of discomfort: effective for back pain.
- Use distraction: playing music, watching TV, and talking on the phone.
- Guided imagery refocuses attention to pleasant thoughts.
- Teach focal point/meditation with concentration on focal point during contractions.
- Encourage use of learned breathing patterns; be aware that some breathing patterns can cause hyperventilation (especially those used during the transition period).
- Use hypnosis, acupressure, therapeutic touch, biofeedback, and aromatherapy, if trained to do so.
- Encourage relaxation and paced breathing.
- Use hydrotherapy (whirlpool, shower) if available.

- Positioning and frequent position changes increase comfort during labor. The woman may assume any position that is comfortable, as a rule; however, supine position should be avoided; lateral position is preferred because it promotes optimal uteroplacental and renal blood flow, and increased fetal oxygen saturation.
- Squatting may be encouraged in second stage labor.
- Sitting, semi-sitting, and lithotomy positions with legs flexed to abdomen also are used in second stage.
- Birthing chair simulates sitting and squatting.
- Kneeling while leaning forward on knees can rotate fetal head.

Critical Thinking Exercise: Nursing Management of the Client with Pain: Nonpharmacologic

Situation: A.F. is a 20-year-old woman, G2 P1, who is in active labor when she comes to the birthing unit. She says that she did not attend childbirth preparation classes during either pregnancy. She does not have insurance and says that she wants to use as little medication as possible in order to keep the cost as low as possible. She is becoming quite uncomfortable, at times moaning during her contractions. The unit does not have a Jacuzzi or tub for a water bath; however, there is a shower in each labor room.

1. Consider two strategies that could be suggested to A.F./partner to break the cycle between fear and tension and then between tension and pain.

2. A.F. chooses the shower for an hour, which her partner with your help/coaching uses to decrease her back pain (shower head pointed to her back) and in different positions (alternating between standing and sitting). You check her frequently and assess her fetal heart rate. A vaginal examination determines that she is now 7-8 cm. and beginning to feel some rectal pressure. What strategies would you include now to decrease fear? Decrease pain?

Nursing Management of the Client with Pain: Pharmacologic Analgesia

> ## Key Points
>
> - Systemic analgesics (e.g., narcotics) work in the central nervous system to decrease the perception of pain.
> - Systemic analgesics cross the placental barrier; given too close to delivery, they can cause respiratory depression in the neonate.
> - The narcotic antagonist, naloxone (Narcan) is used to reverse neonatal narcosis.
> - The intravenous route is preferred for systemic analgesics in labor.
> - Drugs used to provide regional analgesia commonly end with the suffix "-caine" (e.g., lidocaine).
> - The "-caine" drugs are sometimes combined with narcotics for epidural administration.
> - For regional analgesics/anesthetics, ensure an adequate fluid volume and monitor blood pressure.
> - **Key Terms/Concepts**: Fear-tension-pain syndrome, systemic analgesics, regional analgesia

Overview

The fear-tension-pain syndrome is a series of client responses to pain: As pain increases, so do fear and anxiety, which become a vicious cycle because an anxious client has heightened perception of painful stimuli. Fear-tension-pain may cause the client to hyperventilate, to cry out, writhe, scream, and/or be unable to follow instructions. Pharmacologic treatment uses medication to relieve or reduce pain. Pain management reduces stress and anxiety, and produces maximum relief while maintaining maximum safety for woman and fetus. There are three types of pharmacologic pain management: systemic, regional, and general.

Risk Factors for Pain

- Fear
- Anxiety
- Fatigue
- Pain cycle
- Uterine/birth canal stretching in labor
- Individual pain tolerance variations
- Malposition of the fetus
- Cephalopelvic disproportion (CPD)

Causes of Labor Pain

First stage labor pain is a result of uterine contractions, stretching of the uterus, and dilating and effacing the cervical os. Fetal presentation may add to the discomfort, as in a posterior presentation. Discomfort is typically in the back and radiates to the abdomen.

Second stage labor pain results in extreme pressure on the perineum and the muscles of the vagina as the fetus pushes forward. Second stage uterine contractions increase in intensity, frequency, and duration.

Third stage labor pain occurs as uterine contractions expel the placenta.

Signs and Symptoms of Pain

- Increased blood pressure
- Tachycardia
- Behavioral manifestations
- Fatigue
- Crying, screaming
- Hyperventilation
- Moaning
- Inability to follow instructions
- Writhing
- Withdrawal or avoidance behaviors

Therapeutic Nursing Management

- Pharmacologic pain relief in labor may involve the administration of:
  - **Narcotic analgesics** (morphine, Demerol, Sublimaze, Nubain, Stadol)—decrease the sensation of pain, or pain perception, without loss of consciousness. During labor, they are usually administered intravenously. Ideally, birth should occur <1 hour or >4 hours after intravenous injection of a narcotic, in order to minimize neonatal CNS depression. Monitor maternal blood pressure, pulse, oxygen saturation, and respirations after administration. Alternatively, patient controlled analgesia (PCA) is an option for women in labor. A basal rate may be set for labor or the woman may be given the option of frequent boluses that are time-limited to provide pain relief.
  - **Barbiturates** (Seconal, Nembutal, Luminal)—used infrequently to relieve anxiety and induce sleep in prodromal or early latent labor
  - **Ataractics** (Sparine, Phenergan, Vistaril)—tranquilizers, used to potentiate analgesics and reduce anxiety
  - **Regional analgesics/anesthetics** (Lidocaine, Novocaine)—produce some pain relief and motor block (whereas anesthesia provides total pain relief and motor block). "Blocks" provide temporary interruption of the conduction of pain impulses in a particular area of the body. It is important to monitor maternal blood pressure because the "-caine" drugs can cause severe hypotension in pregnant women.

- **The primary nursing responsibility** when administering pain relief medications is to monitor maternal and fetal well-being. This includes monitoring fetal heart rate and maternal vital signs, especially respirations, oxygen saturation, and blood pressure. Assessing for pain relief and effectiveness of pharmaceuticals is critical to this intervention.

Complications

- All forms of pain medications cross the placental barrier and must be given correctly to prevent maternal/fetal complications.
- Pharmacologic agents can cause changes in fetal heart rate/pattern and respiratory depression in the neonate and the mother.
- Narcotic analgesics may cause respiratory depression in the neonate.
- Epidural analgesics/anesthetics may cause a maternal hypotension.
- Narcan, an opioid antagonist is required for neonatal resuscitation and critical for women who have been given analgesia during labor for respiratory depression in the newborn. Not all newborns will require this but it should be present in the emergency equipment at the birth.

Critical Thinking Exercise: Nursing Management of the Client with Pain: Pharmacologic Analgesia

Situation: J.T., G2 P1, is in active labor. Her cervix is dilated to 5 cm. She is experiencing a great deal of anxiety and pain and is unable to stay in control and breathe through her contractions. She does not want an epidural, so the primary care provider has prescribed morphine by PCA pump.

1. What benefits are there to J.T. to have medication in this form?

2. How soon can J.T. expect some relief from her pain?

3. What observations are important for the nurse to make after giving the medications?

4. Because of the side effects of these medications, what nursing diagnosis is needed in order to plan safety measures for J.T.?

5. What important nursing interventions are needed to address this nursing diagnosis?

6. What contraindications are there to use of a PCA pump in labor?

Nursing Management of the Client with Pain: Anesthesia

Key Points

- Spinal anesthesia is inserted into the subarachnoid space; it is used for cesarean births, primarily.
- Epidural anesthesia is injected into the epidural space.
- An intravenous line and a preadministration bolus of intravenous fluid are used prior to regional nerve blocks, to expand the blood volume and prevent hypotension.
- Important maternal assessments after regional blocks: blood pressure, respirations, sensation in, and ability to move legs
- Observe fetal heart rate and variability.
- Continue to monitor labor progress (uterine contractions and cervical dilation).
- General anesthesia is rarely used for childbirth, except when rapid anesthesia is needed in an emergency situation.
- **Key Terms/Concepts**: Analgesia, anesthesia, local anesthesia, regional anesthesia, general anesthesia

Overview

Anesthesia relieves pain by producing loss of sensation and either motor block or loss of consciousness. Local, regional, or general anesthesia may be used. A variety of compounds are used to produce local and regional anesthesia, most are related chemically to cocaine and end with the suffix "caine" (lidocaine, bupivacaine, chloroprocaine).

Types of Local and Regional Anesthesia

Pudendal block: May be used in late second stage to produce light perineal anesthesia for delivery.

Paracervical block: Given intravaginally into the cervix during active first stage labor. Provides local pain relief at the cervix.

Spinal block: Injected directly into spinal canal in late second stage labor. Peaks immediately and lasts up to six hours. Woman must lie flat for the first six hours postpartum to avoid spinal headache.

Epidural block: Injected into epidural space outside the spinal canal, using a flexible catheter when the cervix is dilated four to six cm. Provides continuous pain relief throughout labor and delivery. May be given by intermittent injections or continuous infusion (via pump) through an indwelling epidural catheter.

General anesthesia: Systemic; administered at time of delivery or just before; used only for complications of delivery; produces unconsciousness.

Complications

- **Pudendal blocks** and local infiltrations have no known side effects.
- **Paracervical and epidural blocks** carry a high risk of maternal hypotension, fetal bradycardia, and fetal distress.
- **Spinal block** carries the risk of maternal hypotension, fetal hypoxia. It also produces post-administration headache in some clients.
- **General anesthesia** produces unconsciousness and lack of client participation in labor and delivery, high risk of circulatory and respiratory depression in fetus, and maternal aspiration.

Therapeutic Nursing Management

- Assess the degree of pain and the effectiveness of treatment.
- The nurse will need to help the woman assume and maintain the position for insertion of the spinal or epidural catheter.
- Assess fetal heart rate during and after pain medication.
- Observe for maternal hypotension and respiratory depression.
- Because the woman with an epidural block, for example, cannot feel her contractions, the nurse must instruct when to bear down during vaginal birth. The client should be monitored every five minutes for hypotension. If the client's blood pressure falls, nursing interventions for hypotension should be initiated immediately. These include increasing the IV rate per protocol, placing her on her left side, administering oxygen. Her legs can also be elevated. The physician should be notified and preparations to administer an IV vasopressor such as phedrine should be made.
- The client with a regional block may be unable to move her legs during labor: assist in position changes, offer bedpan for voiding, and observe for urinary retention.
- After the client has a regional block, keep side rails up and place call bell within reach when the nurse is not present.
- Be sure there is no prolonged pressure on any anesthetized part (e.g., do not place client in lateral position with one leg on top of the other unless you put a pillow between the legs).
- For a client with regional anesthesia, pad stirrups for delivery and use care in placing the legs into them simultaneously.
- Prior to standing after delivery, the nurse must determine that sensation has returned to legs/feet. Assist the client with standing/walking until determining that the client can do so safely.

Critical Thinking Exercise: Nursing Management of the Client with Pain: Anesthesia

Situation: A 30-year-old woman is in active labor. She is a gravida 3, TPAL: 1011. Her cervix is dilated to 6 cm and is completely effaced. Her membranes are intact. She is complaining of pain with her uterine contractions (an eight on a scale of zero to ten)and is asking for an epidural.

1. What are the advantages of having an epidural block (as compared with a systemic narcotic analgesic)?

2. What are the disadvantages of having an epidural block?

3. Why is a spinal anesthetic most often used for Cesarean births?

4. This client has a nursing diagnosis of pain related to processes of labor. What are appropriate outcomes for this diagnosis?

5. What important nursing interventions performed prior to the insertion of the epidural can prevent hypotension and fetal bradycardia?

Nursing Management of the Client Requiring Fetal Heart Rate Monitoring

Key Points

- Electronic fetal monitoring is used to evaluate fetal well-being in both the antepartum and intrapartum stages.
- The fetal heart rate (FHR) can be monitored externally or internally.
- Normal FHR is 110-160 beats per minute according to the AACOG standards.
- If the FHR pattern indicates fetal distress, the nurse should:
  - Reposition client to side-lying.
  - Elevate head of bed to 30 degrees.
  - Discontinue intravenous oxytocin.
  - Administer oxygen by facemask at eight to 10 L/min.
  - Notify the primary care provider immediately.
- **Key Terms/Concepts**: Variability, accelerations, decelerations, late decelerations

Overview

Electronic fetal monitoring is used during pregnancy to monitor fetal status. The monitor records the fetal heart rate (FHR) graphically to ensure fetal well-being and placental functioning. Continuous electronic fetal monitoring during labor provides evidence to identify the fetus in danger of asphyxia. The health care team should intervene appropriately to relieve maternal distress. The fetal monitor may be applied externally or internally. An ultrasound transducer and a tocodynamometer are applied to the client's abdomen in external monitoring. Internal fetal monitoring is accomplished through application of a fetal spiral electrode through the birth canal onto the fetus (membranes must be ruptured). The normal fetal heart rate is 110-160 beats per minute.

Factors that Indicate Use of Fetal Monitors

- Abnormal contraction stress test
- Multiple gestation
- Placenta previa
- Oxytocin infusion
- Fetal bradycardia
- Maternal complications (e.g., diabetes, pregnancy-induced hypertension, renal disease)
- Intrauterine growth retardation

- Post dates
- Meconium-stained fluid
- Abruptio placenta, suspected or actual

Signs and Symptoms

Accelerations are an increase in the FHR of 10-15 beats per minute, lasting 10-15 seconds. A healthy fetus with an adequately-functioning placenta will have an acceleration in heart rate in response to movement, so this is a reassuring sign.

Decelerations are a decrease in the fetal heart rate for a short period of time. **Late decelerations** occur after the contraction begins and continue until after the contraction is over. They suggest placental insufficiency and fetal anoxia.

Variability is the normal irregularity in fetal cardiac rhythm. It is seen on the monitor strip as a jagged, irregular (rather than smooth) line. Average or moderate variability is a reassuring sign. Absent or minimal variability is concerning.

Therapeutic Nursing Management

Nurses are responsible for identifying and interpreting changes in FHR patterns. When the FHR pattern is not reassuring, (e.g., loss of variability, late or variable decelerations) the following interventions may be indicated, depending on the nature of the problem:

- Reposition client to side-lying.
- Elevate head of bed to 30 degrees.
- Discontinue intravenous oxytocin.
- Administer oxygen by facemask at 8 to 10 L/min.
- Notify the primary care provider immediately.

Complications

- Some clients find continuous monitoring during labor restrictive/constricting.
- Internal monitoring increases the potential for infection and hemorrhage.
- Internal monitoring requires rupture of membranes and cervical dilation.
- Internal FHR monitoring can be done without internal monitoring of uterine activity.

Critical Thinking Exercise: Nursing Management of the Client Requiring Fetal Heart Rate Monitoring

Situation: : A woman is in active labor at 41 weeks + five days with an oxytocin induction. Her cervix is dilated to four cm and her membranes are intact. The FHR and uterine contractions are being monitored by an external electronic fetal monitor. The nurse notes a fetal heart rate of 110 beats per minute with average variability. There are no decelerations, but there are occasional accelerations up to a rate of 135/minute that last for 30 seconds.

1. Which data should be interpreted as positive signs?

2. One hour later, the only change in the monitor strip is that the FHR variability has decreased and is now described as "minimal." The woman is describing contractions that are increasing in strength but due to her size (>250 lb), it is difficult to assess her contractions. An internal fetal scalp electrode would be beneficial in assessing her uterine activity. What must occur prior to its insertion?

3. After the internal fetal scalp electrode is placed, you note that her contractions are frequent (>5 in 10 minutes) and now there are variable decelerations that occur with each contraction. What actions would be appropriate at this time?

Leopold's Maneuvers

Key Points

- Leopold's maneuvers are used to determine fetal position, lie, presentation, attitude, descent, and presenting part.
- The FHR is heard best directly over the fetal back, which is located during Leopold's maneuvers.
- Have the woman empty her bladder before beginning.
- Position the client on her back for this procedure (may use a wedge under one hip to prevent supine hypotension)–but briefly.
- If you are right-handed, stand on the woman's right, facing her.
- Auscultate fetal heart tones when finished.
- **Key Terms/Concepts**: Leopold's maneuvers, fetal heart rate, client teaching

Overview

Leopold's maneuvers involve external palpation of the client's uterus to determine the number of fetuses; the presenting part, fetal lie, and fetal attitude; the amount of descent into the pelvis; and the expected location for auscultating the fetal heart sounds on the woman's abdomen.

Leopold's Maneuvers

- Face the client; place both hands on the client's abdomen, cupping hands around the fundus. Palpate the part that occupies the fundus. This helps identify fetal lie and presentation. A firm, rounded mass in the fundus is indicative of a vertex fetal presentation.
- Move your hands to either side of the fundus. Hold one hand steady–apply pressure to the fetus. Palpate the fetal back and the irregularities that identify the hands, feet, and elbows. This helps identify presentation.
- Use thumb and middle finger to palpate just above the symphysis pubis. Palpate for the fetal presenting part. If the head is the presenting part, determine the attitude (flexed or extended).
- Face client's feet and palpate both sides of abdomen to determine cephalic prominence. This helps identify descent, attitude, and presentation. Use the flat palmar surfaces of the fingers to do the Leopold's maneuver. Use gentle, firm pressure.

Therapeutic Nursing Management

- Ask the woman to empty her bladder before the assessment.
- Position her supine with one pillow under her head and with her knees slightly flexed.
- Place small, rolled towel under her right hip to displace uterus to the left and prevent supine hypotension.
- Upon completion of Leopold's maneuvers, the nurse should auscultate fetal heart tones to assess for tolerance of the procedure and potential change in fetal position.
- Fetal heart rate is best heard by Doppler over the fetus' back.

Critical Thinking Exercise: Leopold's Maneuvers

Situation: A woman has just been admitted to the assessment area (triage) of the birthing unit. The nurse has taken her vital signs and has completed a brief general systems review. The nurse now intends to perform Leopold's maneuvers as part of her assessment.

1. What information can the nurse obtain by doing Leopold's maneuvers?

2. What should the nurse do before actually palpating the woman's abdomen?

3. How many times should the nurse perform this procedure during the labor? Would all of the maneuvers be complete with each assessment?

4. What should the nurse do after completing the procedure?

5. Which women may be challenging in terms of performing this assessment?

Nursing Management of the Client with Rupture of Membranes (ROM)

Key Points

- Normal amniotic fluid is pale, straw-colored, thin, watery, and without strong odor.
- ROM may occur with a small trickle or a gush of fluid from the vagina.
- ROM can be confirmed by using Nitrazine paper to check the pH of the fluid.
- Prolonged ROM, more than 12-24 hours before birth, predisposes the client and fetus to infection.
- **Key Terms/Concepts:** Spontaneous rupture of membranes (SROM), artificial rupture of membranes (AROM), premature rupture of membranes (PROM), amniotomy

Overview

The main function of the amniotic fluid is to cushion and protect the fetus. Rupture of membranes produces a gush or trickle of amniotic fluid from the vagina when the amniotic membranes tear or give way. This leakage is uncontrollable, and is differentiated from urine by testing for pH with Nitrazine paper. Membranes can rupture spontaneously before or at any time during labor.

Premature, preterm, prolonged rupture of membranes: (PPPROM) is the spontaneous rupture of the membranes before the onset of labor, before 37 weeks gestation, and for greater than 24 hours.

Leopold's Maneuvers

- Characteristics of normal amniotic fluid
- Color—pale and straw colored
- Viscosity—thin and watery
- Odor—no strong odor
- Volume—500-1200 mL

Signs and Symptoms

- Trickle or gush of clear fluid from vaginal area
- Some women mistake leaking or rupture of membranes for incontinence.

Diagnostic Tests and Lab

- **Nitrazine paper:** Nitrazine paper will turn blue if alkaline amniotic fluid (pH 6.5-7.5) is detected.

- **Ferning**: A small amount of amniotic fluid placed on a slide and viewed under a microscope displays a characteristic frond-like pattern called "ferning".

Therapeutic Nursing Management

- Assist with **amniotomy** if necessary (artificial rupture of membranes [AROM] performed by the primary care provider).
- Immediately upon ROM, document the time, appearance, odor, and amount of fluid, and monitor the FHR.
- The umbilical cord may prolapse when membranes rupture; monitor the FHR for several minutes immediately upon ROM to assure fetal well-being.
- If there are abnormal findings (e.g., meconium-stained fluid), institute continuous fetal monitoring and notify primary care provider.
- If premature rupture of membranes occurs:
  - Monitor for signs of premature labor.
  - Observe for prolapsed cord.
  - Prevent exposure to infection–no vaginal exams, etc.
  - Monitor temperature, FHT, contractions.
  - Maintain bed rest as ordered.
  - Administer antibiotics as ordered.
  - Instruct the client about signs and symptoms of infection.

Complications

Infection: Prolonged rupture more than 12-24 hours before birth predisposes client to infection. Infection is suspected if fluid is thick, cloudy, or foul smelling.

Fetal distress: May be indicated by greenish-brown, yellow-stained, or port-wine colored fluid.

Prolapsed cord: Protrusion of the umbilical cord into the vagina ahead of the presenting part. If cord is positioned between the bony pelvis and the fetal presenting part, it becomes compressed and the fetus becomes anoxic. THIS IS A TRUE OBSTETRICAL EMERGENCY.

Critical Thinking Exercise: Nursing Management of the Client with Rupture of Membranes (ROM)

Situation: Elise arrives at the birthing center after being in labor for six hours. Her cervix is dilated to four cm and she is having mild contractions, occurring every five to ten minutes and lasting for 50-60 seconds. The external monitor shows a FHR of 130 bpm, with moderate variability. When her membranes rupture, the fluid is heavily stained with meconium.

1. How would you describe this to her as a first sign of labor?

2. How would the nurse explain the meconium-stained fluid to Elise/partner?

3. What nursing assessments would the nurse include in her care when the membranes ruptured?

4. What initial preparations would the nurse include in her equipment for this baby's birth?

5. Two hours later, her cervix is dilated only to 5 cm. Her contractions are still only mild-to-moderate and of the same frequency and duration. The decision is made to stimulate her labor with oxytocin (Pitocin). What would be the rationale for this decision?

Nursing Management of the Client with Preterm Labor

Key Points

- Tocolytics act by depressing smooth muscle; that is also the source of some of their side effects.
- Nursing care consists of monitoring FHR and uterine contractions, providing emotional support, and monitoring and managing the side effects of tocolytic medications.
- Symptoms of preterm labor: cramping and vaginal discharge
- If symptoms occur at home, advise the woman to:
  - Lie on her left side for 1 hour and drink 2-3 glasses of water.
  - Call or go to the hospital if symptoms continue.
- If symptoms occur at home, advise the woman to call the care provider immediately if she has:
  - Contractions every 5 minutes or less
  - Vaginal bleeding
  - Odorous vaginal discharge
  - Fluid leaking from her vagina
- **Key Terms/Concepts:** Preterm labor, preterm birth, tocolytics, antenatal glucocorticoids, magnesium sulfate, beta-andrenergic antagonists, calcium channel blockers

Overview

Preterm labor is the onset of regular contractions resulting in dilation and effacement of the cervix prior to 20 and 37 weeks of gestation. Preterm birth is a birth that occurs before the end of 37 weeks gestation. The incidence of preterm birth in the U.S. is 10%. Preterm labor accounts for most perinatal deaths not caused by congenital anomalies. Preterm infants have 120 times greater chance of neonatal mortality than term (40 wk) infants. Clients with preterm labor are advised to restrict their activities and avoid sexual intercourse, and may even be placed on bed rest with increased hydration. Tocolytic therapy may be used to delay the birth long enough for antenatal glucocorticoids to be given to accelerate fetal lung maturity.

Risk Factors

- Prior preterm delivery
- Drug or alcohol abuse
- Low socioeconomic status
- Age: Under 20 and over 40 years

- Prior history of abortions
- Poor nutrition
- Smoking
- Heavy or stressful work
- Lack of prenatal care
- Multiple gestations
- Hydramnios
- Abdominal surgery during pregnancy
- Urinary tract infections
- Chorioamnionitis

Signs and Symptoms

There are seven warning signs of preterm labor:

- Regular uterine contractions or occurring every 10 minutes (or more often); may occur with or without pain
- Intestinal cramping, with or without diarrhea
- Menstrual-like cramps
- Low backache
- Pelvic pressure
- Increase or change in vaginal discharge
- Premature rupture of membranes

Diagnostic Tests

- **Electronic fetal monitoring**: Women suspected of preterm labor are monitored using an electronic fetal monitor. Diagnosis of preterm labor is made when uterine contractions are documented at 4 in 20 minutes or 8 in 60 minutes, accompanied by cervical effacement of 80% or dilation of 2 cm or more.

Therapeutic Nursing Management

- Assess for ruptured membranes.
- Assess uterine contractions for frequency, duration, regularity, and intensity.
- Administer tocolytic medications, explain the purposes, and monitor for side effects.
- If receiving tocolytic therapy, assess vital signs regularly; notify provider if maternal pulse exceeds 120.
- If receiving tocolytic therapy, assess for pulmonary edema (chest pain, shortness of breath, crackles, rhonchi).
- If receiving tocolytic therapy, monitor urinary output hourly; monitor for ketonuria.
- If receiving tocolytic therapy, limit fluid intake (usually to 2500-3000 mL/day).
- If receiving magnesium sulfate, monitor respirations, blood pressure, reflexes, and level of consciousness.

- Monitor electrolytes and blood glucose levels.
- Maintain client on bed rest in left lateral position.
- Maintain hydration orally or through intravenous fluids.
- Administer sedation and maintain appropriate safety measures.

If client is at home, advise her to:

- Maintain bed rest until symptoms subside.
- Drink two to three glasses of water or juice.
- Call the care provider if symptoms return.
- Avoid sexual intercourse.
- Call the care provider immediately if she has:
  - Contractions every 5 minutes or less
  - Vaginal bleeding
  - Odorous vaginal discharge
  - Fluid leaking from her vagina

Pharmacology

- Administer antenatal glucocorticoids to accelerate fetal lung maturity, usually prior to 34 weeks gestation.
- Administer tocolytic drugs to suppress uterine activity. The following are most often used:
  - Beta-adrenergic antagonists (ritodrine, terbutaline)—relax uterine muscle. They may be administered intravenously, subcutaneously, or orally.
  - Magnesium sulfate—administered intravenously to depress uterine contractility. It is safer than ritodrine or terbutaline.
  - Calcium channel blockers (Procardia)
  - Prostaglandin inhibitors (indomethacin, NSAIDs such as naproxen, and salicylates)

Complications

- Side effects of tocolytic medications (beta mimetics)
  - Tachycardia
  - Dysrhythmias
  - Pulmonary edema
  - Altered glucose metabolism
  - Tremors
  - Hypokalemia
  - Fetal tachycardia (magnesium sulfate)
  - Respiratory depression
  - Hypotension
  - Central nervous system depression, including depressed reflexes; and level of consciousness

- Physiologic complications related to preterm birth:
  - Respiratory distress
  - Hyperbilirubinemia

Critical Thinking Exercise: Nursing Management of the Client with Preterm Labor

Situation: A 42-year-old woman in the 34th week of pregnancy is admitted to the birthing unit assessment area because she is experiencing contractions. She is gravida 4, para 0; previous pregnancies have ended in miscarriage or preterm birth. Her cervix is dilated to 2-3 cm; uterine contractions are occurring every five to ten minutes. She says, "I can feel the contractions, but they aren't painful." Electronic fetal monitoring, intravenous (IV) magnesium sulfate, and bed rest are ordered. Betamethasone (a glucocorticoid) is also ordered and is to be given intramuscularly (IM) immediately and repeated in 12 hours.

1. What risk factors does this woman have for preterm labor?

2. What assessments would the nurse in the assessment (triage) area of the birthing unit include in her care?

3. What other symptoms of preterm labor are important for the nurse to assess? Why?

4. What are contraindications or cautions for betamethasone therapy?

5. How should the nurse prioritize these interventions? (a) Start the IV and begin administering the magnesium sulfate, (b) apply the external fetal monitor, (c) administer the betamethasone IM, (d) explain the need for bed rest and the other interventions. Explain your reasoning.

6. In general, how would this woman's care be different if she were at 22 weeks gestation?

Nursing Management of the Client with an Episiotomy

Key Points

- Potential complications: Pain, infection, and hematoma
- Prevention: Apply ice pack to perineum immediately after birth to minimize edema and pain.
- Comfort: Sitz bath, witch hazel pads, oral analgesics
- Teaching: Perineal hygiene ("front-to-back"), signs/symptoms of infection
- **Key Terms/Concepts**: Episiotomy, laceration, perineum, median episiotomy, mediolateral episiotomy, REEDA

Overview

An episiotomy is a surgical incision of the perineum to enlarge the vaginal outlet. Proponents of using the episiotomy say that it prevents perineal lacerations, minimizes stretching of perineal muscles (helping to prevent later stress incontinence), reduces duration of the second stage, and makes it easier to perform manipulations (e.g., forceps or vacuum extraction) to facilitate the infant's birth. Opponents of the procedure say that lacerations may occur even with an episiotomy, and that the pain and healing time are greater than that associated with lacerations. Alternative measures for perineal management include: preparing for birth through using Kegel exercises and massage in the prenatal period; using squatting or lateral positions during birth in order to allow for gradual stretching of the perineal tissues; use of warm compresses, manual support, and massage.

Risk Factors for Perineal Trauma (Episiotomy or Lacerations)

- Nulliparity
- Occiput posterior fetal position
- Large fetus
- Use of instruments (e.g., forceps or vacuum)
- Fetal distress
- Prolonged second stage

Types of Episiotomy

Median: Down the midline. This is the most commonly used type.

Mediolateral: A 30° angle from the midline. Blood loss is greater and it is more painful than the median episiotomy, but it allows for more room in operative births.

Therapeutic Nursing Management (Recovery and Postpartum Period)

- Apply ice pack to perineum/episiotomy immediately after birth (12-24 hours).
- Inspect during every shift to determine condition/healing.
- Provide comfort measures: Tucks or witch hazel pads.
- Provide sitz bath (after 12-24 hours).
- Teach client that healing should be complete in 3-4 weeks and sutures are dissolving.
- Instruct about signs and symptoms of infection.
- Instruct about proper hygiene regarding pad changes and after bowel movements.

Complications

- Median episiotomy may "extend" through the anal sphincter during delivery.
- Mediolateral episiotomy is more difficult to repair and more susceptible to healing complications.
- Infection
- Hematoma:
    - Symptoms include those of postpartum hemorrhage plus a firm uterus with bright red blood in vagina.
    - Vulvar hematoma is seen as a bulging, bluish swelling that is painful to palpation.
    - Vaginal or peritoneal hematoma are harder to diagnose.
    - Management:
        - Depends on early diagnosis and treatment to prevent morbidity and mortality
        - Complaints of severe pain in perineal or rectal region in early puerperium require examination for hematoma.
        - Usually are small and result in minimal sequelae
        - Treated with ice packs and analgesics
        - If hematoma expands or becomes very large, surgical evacuation is needed; blood transfusions and antibiotics may be needed.
- Delayed healing
- Increased blood loss
- Scarring
- Increased pain
- Sexual dysfunction
- Higher costs because of time and suturing
- Physiologic complications related to preterm birth:
    - Respiratory distress
    - Hyperbilirubinemia

Critical Thinking Exercise: Nursing Management of the Client with an Episiotomy

Situation: D.D. has come to the pre-admission clinic with her birth plan. She is gravida 1 TPAL: 0000. She has written on her plan that she does not want to have an episiotomy.

1. As the pre-admission nurse, how would you begin your discussion with D.D. and her partner regarding episiotomy?

2. What would you suggest to D.D. that she could do antenatally to prevent an episiotomy?

Situation: D.D. is now in second stage labor. The fetus is quite large and the fetal monitor is showing early signs of fetal distress. As D.D. has already been in second stage labor for quite a while, it seems likely that she will need an episiotomy even though she has said that she would prefer not to have one.

3. What strategies might the nurse use to try and help D.D. achieve her goal of an intact perineum?

4. If the physician or midwife determines that an episiotomy is required, what nursing measures will be needed postpartum?

Nursing Management of the Client with Forceps-Assisted Birth

Key Points

- Determination of the need for forceps-assisted birth is a medical decision.
- Intrapartum Nursing Interventions:
    - Explain activities to the client.
    - Be sure the client's bladder is empty.
    - Monitor the fetal heart rate.
    - Report to newborn and postpartum caregivers that forceps were used at birth.
- Postpartum Nursing Interventions:
    - Assess the mother for vaginal and cervical lacerations and bladder injuries.
    - Assess the neonate for bruising, facial palsy, and subdural hematoma
- **Key Terms/Concepts**: Low forcep, midforcep, labial-vaginal hematoma

Overview

During the second stage of labor, it may be necessary to facilitate delivery when maternal efforts are insufficient. Obstetric forceps are used to provide traction, rotation, or both to the fetal head to aid in the expulsion of the fetus. Forceps are similar to two large metal tongs, separated and applied one at a time to each side of the fetal head. Forceps deliveries are classified according to the level and position of the fetal head relative to the pelvic outlet. Low forceps control the head after it is visible at the vaginal outlet. Mid forceps are applied when the fetal head is +2 station or higher.

Maternal Indications for a Forceps-Assisted Delivery

- Prolonged labor
- Limited maternal reserve
- Maternal exhaustion
- Maternal illness

Fetal Indications for a Forceps-Assisted Birth

- Fetal distress
- Fetal malpresentation
- Large fetal head

Conditions Necessary for Successful Forceps-Assisted Birth

- Cervix fully dilated—to avert lacerations and hemorrhage
- Bladder empty

- Presenting part is engaged
- Vertex is presenting (as a rule)
- Membranes are ruptured
- Cephalopelvic disproportion (CPD) is not present

Therapeutic Nursing Management

- Obtain the specified forceps.
- Be sure that the woman's bladder is empty; catheterize if necessary.
- Check, report, and record fetal heart rate (FHR) before forceps are applied.
- Check FHR after forceps are applied. If a drop occurs, they would be removed and reapplied.
- Once the forceps are applied, the nurse should monitor contractions (traction is applied during contractions).
- After birth, assess mother for vaginal and cervical lacerations (evidenced by bleeding) and bladder retention, which may indicate bladder injury.
- Assess infant for bruising or abrasions at the site of blade application, facial palsy, and subdural hematoma. Document the size and location in the infant's medical record.

Complications

- Laceration and bruising may occur to the woman's vagina and cervix, or the episiotomy may extend into the rectal tissue, putting the client at greater risk for infection.
- The neonate may have head or face bruising, subdural hematoma, or facial palsy.
- Severe complications include subarachnoid hemorrhage, and less commonly, intracranial hemorrhage or skull fracture.

Critical Thinking Exercise: Nursing Management of the Client with Forceps-Assisted Birth

Situation: T.J. is in labor. She is gravida 1 para 0. Her cervix is fully dilated, membranes are ruptured and, contractions are strong. T.J. has been pushing with the contractions with little progress (descent). The fetus is engaged and in vertex position. The fetus is quite large and the fetal monitor is showing that the fetal heart rate is non-reassuring. The primary care provider has indicated that he/she has decided to do a forceps-assisted birth. When T. J. sees the forceps, she is afraid. She says, "Please be careful. You could crush my baby's head with those things!"

1. What nursing assessments should be made before the forceps are used?

2. Specifically, why must the nurse check, report, and record the FHR both before and after application of the forceps?

3. What indicators are in place to facilitate the use of forceps?

4. How will the health care provider likely describe the need for forceps in this situation?

Nursing Management of the Client with Vacuum-Assisted Birth

> ## Key Points
>
> - Determination of the need for vacuum-assisted birth is a medical decision.
> - Intrapartum Nursing Interventions:
>   - Explain activities to the client.
>   - Place client in lithotomy position.
>   - Monitor the fetal heart rate.
>   - Report to newborn and postpartum caregivers that vacuum extraction was used.
> -
>   - Assess the neonate for trauma at application site.
>   - Assess the neonate for signs of cerebral irritation (e.g., poor sucking, listlessness).
>   - If bruising or cephalhematoma occur, observe for subsequent jaundice.
> - **Key Terms/Concepts**: Vacuum extraction, neonatal complications, CPD

Overview

Vacuum extraction involves the attachment of a vacuum cup to the fetal head to exert negative pressure; traction is then applied to facilitate descent of the fetal head. The woman is urged to continue to push with contractions. Vacuum extraction is used to shorten the second stage of labor in the event of dystocia, in cases of cardiac decompensation, and in cases of fetal distress. Approximately 7% of births are vacuum-assisted, although that rate is increasing in efforts to reduce the number of surgically-assisted deliveries (cesarean sections). Vacuum extraction is now more widely used than forceps-assisted birth.

Conditions Necessary for Vacuum Extraction

- Vertex presentation
- Absence of cephalopelvic disproportion (CPD)
- Ruptured membranes

Therapeutic Nursing Management

- Place the woman in the lithotomy position.
- Explain the procedure.
- Encourage the woman to push during contractions.
- Assess the FHR frequently during the procedure.

- Observe newborn for trauma at the application site.
- Observe newborn for cephalhematoma.
- Observe newborn for cerebral irritation (e.g., poor suck-swallow, listlessness).
- Observe newborn for jaundice as bruising resolves.
- Reassure parents that caput succedaneum at application site is normal and will begin to disappear within a few hours.
- Report to postpartum and nursery personnel that vacuum extraction was used.

Potential Complications

- Neonatal: Cephalhematoma, scalp lacerations, subdural hematoma
- Maternal (uncommon): Perineal, vaginal, or cervical lacerations

Critical Thinking Exercise: Nursing Management of the Client with Vacuum-Assisted Birth

Situation: M.J. is in second stage labor. She is gravida 1 para 0. Her cervix is fully dilated; the fetus is engaged and in vertex position. The fetus' heart rate has decreased variability in the baseline with variable decelerations. M.J. is very tired as she has been pushing for more than 1.5 hours. She is having trouble focusing and pushing with her contractions. The primary care provider tells M.J. and her partner that he/she will be using a vacuum extractor to assist with the baby's birth.

1. What conditions are present in this situation that have led to the decision to use the vacuum extractor to assist with birth?

2. List five contraindications for vacuum extraction.

3. Prior to the vacuum application, what two maternal assessments should the nurse make?

4. What documentation is critical?

Nursing Management of the Client with Post-term Labor

Key Points

- Risks are primarily to the fetus.
- Maternal risk is associated with delivery of a large baby: birth injuries or the need for cesarean birth.
- Oligohydramnios is common, increasing the risk of fetal cord compression.
- In 20-30% of post-term pregnancies, placental function deteriorates, resulting in fetal hypoxia and malnourishment, and subsequent poor tolerance of labor.
- During labor: observe for FHR decelerations, prepare for emergency birth, and respond to respiratory problems of the newborn.
- Post-term infants have a higher perinatal mortality rate than term infants.
- **Key Terms/Concepts:** Post-term labor, oligohydramnios, placental insufficiency, biophysical profile, amnioinfusion

Overview

A post-term pregnancy is one that extends beyond the 42nd week of gestation, or 294 days from the first day of the last menstrual period. The incidence of post-term pregnancy is about 10%. As the baby may be excessively large, the woman is at risk for dysfunctional labor and lacerations, induction of labor, forceps- or vacuum-assisted birth, and cesarean birth. Accurate determination of the due date is important when evaluating the client for post-term labor.

After the 41st week, the placenta "ages," and its function decreases. If placental insufficiency is present, there are alterations in oxygen and nutrients delivered to the fetus, so the fetus is at risk for fetal distress during labor. Problems may include asphyxia, meconium aspiration, dysmaturity syndrome, and respiratory distress. In addition, amniotic fluid volume declines dramatically between 40 and 42 weeks' gestation, increasing the likelihood of hypoxia resulting from fetal cord compression. Post-term delivery accounts for 15% of neonatal mortality. Women are also usually anxious about going past their estimated due date.

Risk Factors

- Previous post-term delivery
- Estrogen deficiency
- Decrease of placental sulfatase (produces estrogen)
- Decreased adrenal cortical function

Signs and Symptoms

- Pregnancy extending past more than 42 weeks
- Diminished fetal growth
- Oligohydramnios

Diagnostic Tests and Labs

- Non-stress and oxytocin-challenge-contraction stress tests for fetal well-being
- Assessment of amniotic fluid volume
- Amniocentesis or amnioscopy to detect meconium in the amniotic fluid
- Biophysical profile
- Ultrasound
- Weekly cervical checks

Therapeutic Nursing Management

- Prepare client for possible induction of labor using oxytocin and cervical ripening (prostaglandin) gel.
- Prepare client for possible forceps-assisted, vacuum-assisted birth, or cesarean birth.
- Assist with amnioinfusion to restore volume, as indicated.
- Monitor fetal and neonatal status.
- Test infant's blood glucose soon after birth and again in one hour. Our current research- based protocols suggest that the focus should be on feeding infants within one hour, preferably 1/2 hour (all infants, not just post-term) and that the first blood glucose level should be done one hour prior to the next feeding for those infants at risk: >4,000 grams, <2,500 grams, infants of diabetic mothers or those with endocrine disease, preterm infants, and those that are symptomatic.
- Provide early and frequent feedings.
- Monitor newborn's temperature frequently; teach parents how to prevent cold stress; provide extra blankets or radiant warmer, as needed.

Complications

- Fetal acidosis
- Oligohydramnios
- Fetal meconium aspiration
- Neonatal mortality
- Neonatal hypoglycemia
- Neonatal polycythemia and subsequent hyperbilirubinemia
- Neonatal impaired thermoregulation
- Fetal wasting

Critical Thinking Exercise: Nursing Management of the Client with Post-term Labor

Situation: E. S. is in the 42nd week of gestation. Her fundal height is 38 cm. At 41 weeks, her fundal height was 39 cm, and at 40 weeks, it was 40 cm. Her primary care provider considers the pregnancy to be post-term and plans to induce labor. E. S. says, "I guess the baby will be even bigger than we expected. However, that's okay, since he's a boy. He can be a football player." The nurse replies, "Some post-term babies are larger than normal, but some are smaller. It is possible that your baby may not be especially large."

1. Which of the preceding data support the nurse's interpretation of E. S.'s situation?

2. What else could E. S.'s decreasing fundal height indicate?

3. Based on ultrasound scanning, it is determined that E. S. does have oligohydramnios. However, an amnioinfusion is not planned. During labor what assessment will be crucial for the nurse to make?

4. What special precautions should the nurse make for E. S.'s labor and birth?

Situation: Ms. T is a G1 TPAL000 at 41 weeks and 5 days gestation. She has been scheduled for an induction using prostaglandin gel. She has had no signs of labor and is very anxious. She is to come to the birthing center at 0900 hours for the gel insertion but the unit is very busy. It is your responsibility, as the nurse in charge, to call her and inform her that you need her to postpone her arrival for approximately six hours until there is a bed and staff available to care for her. She is extremely upset and tells you that her partner has taken the day off work.

5. What would you include in your information to Ms. T. and her plan of care?

Ms. T. comes in six hours later and prostaglandin gel is inserted as initially planned. Ms. T. has been monitored for one hour as per unit policy. Start a new sentence and replace with; "There were no contractions palpated or noted on the fetal heart rate tracing. The electronic monitor strip was reassuring with no significant fetal heart rate decelerations. Ms. T. is now able to go home overnight and will return in the morning for reassessment and possibly an oxytocin induction.

6. What would you include in your teaching regarding warning signs and symptoms requiring return for assessment earlier than planned and information regarding an oxytocin induction?

Nursing Management of the Client with a Prolapsed Umbilical Cord

Key Points

- Factors that increase the risk for prolapsed cord:
  - Fetal presenting part at high station
  - Small fetus or abnormal presentation (e.g., breech)
  - Hydramnios
- Prolapsed cord cannot always be seen.
- Prolapsed cord is an emergency; birth must be achieved rapidly to prevent fetal asphyxia.
- When prolapse occurs, key interventions are to:
  - Relieve pressure on the cord.
  - Expedite delivery.
  - Call for help, but do not leave the woman.
- **Key Terms/Concepts:** Prolapsed cord, Trendelenburg position, emergency situation

Overview

Prolapse of the umbilical cord occurs when, after rupture of the membranes, the cord slips down into the pelvic outlet ahead of the presenting fetal parts. The fetal presenting part may partially or completely compress the umbilical cord, reducing or stopping blood flow to the fetus. Occult prolapse is hidden, not visible, and can occur at any time in labor whether or not the membranes are ruptured. Visible prolapse usually occurs directly after rupture of membranes, when gravity washes the cord out in front of the presenting part. Prolapsed cord occurs in approximately 1 of 400 births.

A prolapsed cord is an EMERGENCY!

Risk Factors

- Unengaged fetal head during labor
- Rupture of membranes–amniotic fluid may carry a loop of fetal cord into the pelvic outlet
- Prematurity or very small fetus
- Hydramnios
- Multiple fetu ses
- Abnormally long cord (>100 cm)
- Abnormal fetal position (e.g., breech, transverse lie)

Signs and Symptoms

- Palpation or visualization of the cord in the cervix or vagina
- Woman reports feeling the cord when membranes rupture
- Fetal bradycardia, variable or late decelerations, or loss of FHR variability (indications of fetal distress)

Therapeutic Nursing Management

- Call for help!
- Notify primary care provider immediately.
- Assess fetal heart rate immediately following rupture of membranes and again in 15 minutes.
- Reposition client in Trendelenburg or knee-chest position if prolapse is suspected or detected. Alternatively, place the woman in side-lying position with hips elevated on pillows.
- Push presenting part away from the cord by inserting a sterile gloved hand into the vagina.
- Give oxygen at 8-10 liters/minute to increase maternal blood oxygen saturation.
- Prepare the client for cesarean birth if necessary.
- Expect the woman and family to be anxious; remain calm to help decrease their anxiety.
- Keep explanations simple, because anxiety interferes with comprehension.

Complications

- The only maternal risks are those associated with cesarean birth.
- Intrauterine cerebral hypoxia or anoxia.
- Fetal demise (prognosis depends upon the severity and length of time that blood flow through the cord has been impaired).

Critical Thinking Exercise: Nursing Management of the Client with a Prolapsed Umbilical Cord

Situation: You are caring for a woman in labor and you have just assisted her to the bathroom. While on the toilet, she feels a "gush of fluid" and now "feels like something fell out".

1. Prioritize the following nursing interventions for this client. Explain your reasoning.

_____ Place the woman in Trendelenburg or knee-chest position.

_____

_____

_____Use a gloved hand to push the fetal presenting part upward and keep it there until birth.

_____

_____

_____Administer oxygen.

_____

_____

_____Notify the primary care provider Stat.

_____

_____

_____Press or pull the call light for emergency assistance.

_____

_____

_____Inspect the perineum to see if the cord is visible.

_____

_____

_____Assess the fetal heart rate.

_____

_____

Nursing Management of the Client with Multifetal Pregnancy

Key Points

- Twins occur about once in 50 pregnancies; triplets, once in 8,100.
- Multifetal pregnancy increases the risk of both maternal and fetal/neonatal complications.
- Fertility drugs increase the likelihood of multifetal pregnancy.
- Common complications include preterm birth and pregnancy-induced hypertension.
- Cesarean birth is frequently necessary–almost always if there are more than two fetuses.
- During labor (for a vaginal birth) each twin's FHR is monitored separately.
- One neonatal nurse or other specialist should be available to care for each infant.
- **Key Concepts/Terms:** Monozygotic twins, dizygotic twins, hypotonic labor

Overview

When two or more embryos develop in the uterus at the same time, the condition is known as a multiple gestation or multifetal pregnancy. With multifetal pregnancies, the risk of morbidity and mortality is increased throughout the antepartum, intrapartum, and postpartum periods. Multifetal pregnancy is suspected when the uterus is larger than normal for the gestational age. The woman may be very uncomfortable during pregnancy because the oversized uterus may cause shortness of breath, dyspnea, backaches, and pedal edema. A major goal is to prevent preterm labor; therefore, prenatal care should begin early, and more frequent visits are encouraged. The woman is advised early in pregnancy to make lifestyle changes, including: reducing the work week hours, and avoiding standing for long periods.

Risk Factors

- Family history of multiple gestation
- Ovulation-inducing drugs
- Infertility treatment—in vitro fertilization (IVF) and gamete intrafallopian tube transfer (GIFT), and fertility drugs such as Clomid
- Advanced maternal age

Signs and Symptoms

- Identification of two or more fetuses by palpation, ultrasound, fundal height, and heart sounds, etc.

- Auscultation of heart sounds in more than one place
- Elevated fundal height
- Severe nausea and vomiting
- Greater weight gain

Diagnostic Tests and Lab

- Elevated HCG levels
- Elevated alpha fetal protein (AFP)
- Elevated progesterone
- Ultrasound
- Amniocentesis

Therapeutic Nursing Management

- Prepare client for cesarean birth if appropriate (twins/triplets often require cesarean birth).
- Continually monitor fetuses if delivering vaginally.
- Identify each neonate carefully.
- Ensure that resuscitation equipment is ready for each newborn.
- Plan for additional nursing staff to assist with additional babies.
- Advise client to avoid standing for prolonged periods of time (during pregnancy).
- A maternal weight gain of 40-50 lbs should be encouraged for a twin pregnancy. A daily intake of 4000 kcal is recommended.

Complications

- Preterm birth—approximately half of twins are born before 37 weeks.
- Spontaneous abortion
- Intrauterine growth retardation (IUGR) due to space confines
- Congenital abnormalities, placental abnormalities, cord accidents, and twin-to-twin transfusion.
- Maternal pregnancy-induced hypertension (PIH), hydramnios, and anemia
- Dysfunctional labor secondary to uterine overdistension and hypotonicity or malpresentation
- Increased risk of uterine rupture
- Increased risk of postpartum hemorrhage

Critical Thinking Exercise: Nursing Management of the Client with Multifetal Pregnancy

Situation: A woman, gravida 3 para 2, at 20 weeks gestation, has been told that she is carrying twins. Her fundal height is greater than expected for the weeks of gestation. Although she states that she has experienced "quite a bit" of nausea and vomiting, she has gained 20 lbs already. The nurse auscultates a heart rate of 160 for Twin A and a heart rate of 140 for Twin B.

1. Evaluate the fetal heart rates.

2. The woman says, "Can you help me with my diet? I need to find a way to get everything the babies need, but still not take in so many calories. My friend only gained 25 lbs the whole time she was pregnant. I'm going to be too fat if I keep this up!" How should the nurse respond?

3. Which maternal vital sign is especially important to assess in this case? Why?

4. What should the nurse teach this woman about preventing preterm labor?

Situation: Ms. S., at G3 TPAL: 1011, comes in for a regularly scheduled office visit at 32 weeks gestation. She describes fatigue, increased slowness with intermittent backache, increased weight gain, decreased mobility and shortness of breath. She has her 3-year-old with her. The fetal heart rates are 135/145 and you go on to assess her vital signs as well.

5. Place a check mark beside each symptom describing whether it is normal for a multifetal pregnancy or abnormal and merits further assessment.

   Fatigue

   Decreased mobility

   Weight gain of 30 lb. at 32 weeks

   Shortness of breath

   FHR 135/145

   Slight edema in her ankles

   BP 150/100

Ms. S. states that she is having trouble coping with this pregnancy and with her toddler and wonders about community resources for both the last few weeks of pregnancy and for postpartum.

6. What would you tell her?

Nursing Management of the Client Requiring a Cesarean Birth (C-Section)

Key Points

- About 20% of births are cesarean; it is important that clients be prepared for this possibility.
- Cesarean birth is performed for a variety of fetal and maternal complications (e.g., non-reassuring fetal heart rate tracing, dystocia, preeclampsia).
- A cesarean birth may be planned (scheduled) or performed in an emergency situation.
- Having one cesarean birth does not necessarily indicate the need for future births to be cesarean.
- Cesarean births have a higher maternal mortality rate than vaginal births.
- Efforts should be made to include the partner in the birth experience. Regardless of the type of birth, the woman/family should be included in the plan of care for birth.
- Postpartum complications include: infection, reactions to anesthesia, hemorrhage, and embolus
- **Key Terms/Concepts:** Cesarean section, preoperative/postoperative care, CPD

Overview

A cesarean section is a surgical procedure in which birth is accomplished through an incision into the abdomen and uterus. It is considered major abdominal surgery. Two types of incisions may be used: classic (vertical into uterine body) or low (transverse at the mons). Cesarean births (c-sections) are more expensive than vaginal births and require a longer recovery time. The goal of cesarean birth is to preserve the life/health of the mother and the fetus; it may be the best choice for birth when there are maternal or fetal complications. Whether a cesarean birth is planned or unplanned (emergency), failure to give birth to a child in the traditional manner may be a source of grief and negative self-concept to the mother. An emergency cesarean section is usually viewed as a traumatic event. Nursing care following an emergency cesarean section should include reinforcing and explaining the events leading to the operation.

Risk Factors Indications for Cesarean Birth

- High risk pregnancy
- Breech presentation, particularly in primiparous women
- Most common indications: CPD (cephalopelvic disproportion), labor disorders, cord compression, malpresentation, fetal distress, previous c-section, abruptio placenta, third trimester bleeding, sexually transmitted diseases

Diagnostic Tests

- Prenatal testing (non-stress and contraction stress tests)
- Electronic fetal monitoring (EFM)
- Ultrasound
- Fetal scalp blood pH during labor

Therapeutic Nursing Management

Preoperative nursing care

- Teach client regarding early ambulation, coughing, and deep breathing.
- Insert indwelling urinary catheter.
- Shave/cleanse abdomen as indicated by institutional policy.
- Maintain NPO status.
- Start IV and intravenous fluids.
- Administer preoperative medications as ordered.
- Monitor client vital signs and fetal heart rate.
- Alleviate anxiety (especially if the c-section is unplanned).

Intraoperative nursing care

- Assist in positioning the woman on the operating table. Use a wedge, or tilt the table, so that the uterus is displaced about 15° from midline (to help prevent vena caval compression).
- Continue to monitor the FHR until immediately prior to surgery.
- Monitor vital signs during anesthesia.
- Monitor intravenous fluids.

Postoperative nursing care

- Take vital signs per protocol. Phase 1 recovery vital signs include temperature taken on admission and hourly until temperature is 35.5° Centigrade or 95.9° Fahrenheit. BP, pulse, respiratory rate assessed on admission and every 15 minutes. Continuous oxygen saturaton monitor with alarm parameters documented on admission and every 15 minutes. Continuous cardiac monitoring with alarm parameters set, documented on admission.
- Assess lochia and fundal tone, the same as for a vaginal birth.
- Monitor intravenous fluids, rate, and amount.
- Observe abdominal incision for bleeding, approximation, and inflammation.
- Monitor intake and output.
- Observe the urine for blood (indication of surgical trauma to the bladder).
- Medicate for pain/nausea.
- Assist with newborn care in early postpartum.

Complications

- **Maternal**: Hemorrhage, infection, dehiscence, pulmonary embolism, aspiration, urinary tract infection
- **Fetal/neonatal**: Respiratory distress, fetal injury

Critical Thinking Exercise: Nursing Management of the Client Requiring a Cesarean Birth (C-Section)

Situation: R. C., a primigravida, has been in prolonged, active labor. She is becoming exhausted. The primary care provider diagnoses cephalopelvic disproportion (CPD), and preparations are being made for a cesarean birth. R. C. and her partner are very worried about the need for surgery and are asking many questions. She says, "I've never been in a hospital before, much less had surgery." R. C. already has an IV, which was inserted early in her labor. The nurse inserts an indwelling urinary catheter. Waiting until the epidural/spinal is in place prior to inserting the urinary catheter is kinder to the woman.

1. What is the purpose of the indwelling catheter?

2. The nurse makes a nursing diagnosis of "anxiety related to lack of knowledge about procedures and uncertain outcome for self and baby." What nursing interventions might be used to promote family-centered care and decrease anxiety? List at least seven.

3. The nurse positions R. C. in supine position on the operating table, with a small pillow under her head. She secures her legs and arms with safety straps, and applies a grounding pad. Evaluate the nurse's actions. What, if anything, needs to be changed?

4. After the birth, the nurse goes to visit the family. R.C. has many questions about what occurred prior to and during the surgery. How is this debriefing helpful for R.C. and her family?

Nursing Management of the Client with Cephalopelvic Disproportion (CPD)

Key Points

- CPD (also called fetopelvic disproportion) occurs when fetal head size is too large to fit through the maternal pelvis.
- CPD is characterized by a lack of fetal descent in the presence of strong contractions.
- Suspect CPD when labor is prolonged, the presenting part does not engage, and cervical dilation and effacement are slow.
- True CPD necessitates a cesarean birth.
- **Key Terms/Concepts**: Fetal descent, dystocia, X-ray pelvimetry, labor progression (Friedman) curve, trial of labor, pelvic contracture, ultrasound

Overview

Cephalopelvic disproportion (CPD) is a condition in which the fetal head is of a size, shape, or position that it cannot pass through the woman's pelvis. Because of the disproportion, it becomes physically impossible for the fetus to be delivered, so a cesarean birth is necessary. CPD is suspected when the fetal head does not descend even in the presence of strong contractions.

Risk Factors

- Gestational diabetes
- Multiparity
- Fetal malformation
- Shape or size of maternal pelvis
- Shape or position of the fetus' head

Signs and Symptoms

- General lack of cervical change or fetal descent during the active phase of first stage labor
- Dystocia–abnormal labor or failure of labor to progress
- Uncontrollable pushing before complete dilation of cervix

Diagnostic Tests

- **Trial labor**: Attempt at vaginal delivery (when measurements indicate borderline CPD)
- **Ultrasound**: Estimation of fetal size compared to manual pelvic measurements (prior to labor) and computed tomography

- **X-ray pelvimetry**: To visualize pelvic measures
- Use of standard **labor progression curves** (Friedman)

Therapeutic Nursing Management

- Assist client to cope emotionally with cesarean delivery.
- Stress the importance of the safety of the baby.
- Monitor FHR, uterine contractions, and cervical dilation.
- Nursing care during "trial of labor" is similar to that of any labor, except that assessments of cervical dilation and fetal descent are done more often. If progress ceases, a cesarean birth is necessary.
- Report any signs of fetal distress to the caregiver immediately.
- Provide emotional support by keeping the woman/couple informed and explaining procedures.
- Help the woman assume different positions to increase the pelvic diameters (e.g., sitting or squatting, changing from one side to the other, hands-and-knees position).

Complications

Maternal: Exhaustion, postpartum hemorrhage secondary to uterine atony, and infection

Infant: Cord prolapse, birth trauma, fractured clavicle, Erb's palsy, and anoxia

Critical Thinking Exercise: Nursing Management of the Client with Cephalopelvic Disproportion (CPD)

Situation: A woman with borderline CPD is being given a trial of labor. The nurse is closely monitoring her cervical dilation and the uterine contractions.

1. Why is information about both cervical dilation and the uterine contractions essential to making judgments about CPD?

2. What other regular observation must be made in order to determine whether the labor is progressing satisfactorily?

3. After the woman is in a sitting position for a period of time, the nurse helps her to assume a squatting position. The woman's membranes rupture; on vaginal exam, the woman's perineum is observed to be bulging and a small area of the fetal head is visualized. What does this mean?

Situation: Ms. S., a G1, TPAL: 0000, patient has been three to four cm. dilated, 100% effaced and -three station with intact amniotic membranes for the last two hours. She is contracting every five minutes, coping well but is discouraged about her labor progress.

4. What risk factors does Ms. S. have for CPD?

5. What other information might assist with this diagnosis?

6. What strategies might the RN suggest to facilitate progress in labor?

Nursing Management of the Client with Meconium-Stained Amniotic Fluid

Key Points

- Meconium passage in utero may or may not be caused by fetal distress.
- When meconium-stained amniotic fluid is seen during labor, fetal distress must be considered.
- In the presence of meconium staining, poor FHR variability and variable or late decelerations are an ominous sign.
- Suction infant at birth to prevent aspiration of meconium.
- Prepare to care for stressed infant, with possible transfer to intensive care unit
- **Key Terms/Concepts**: Green-tinged amniotic fluid, hypoxia, neonatal complications

Overview

Meconium passed prior to delivery produces a greenish tinge to the amniotic fluid or even heavy particulate matter within the fluid. If the fetus becomes distressed and hypoxic, the anal sphincter relaxes and the fetus expels meconium into the amniotic fluid, staining it green. Presence of meconium before onset of labor does not usually indicate a problem; the fetus may pass meconium even without being stressed, or the stress may have been temporary. When meconium staining is detected during labor, however, electronic fetal monitoring and perhaps fetal scalp blood sampling is necessary to determine fetal well-being. To prevent and detect meconium aspiration in the neonate, the nurse should monitor the fetus more carefully. The newborn's trachea may be visualized and suctioned to prevent meconium aspiration syndrome.

Possible causes of meconium passage:

- A normal physiological function, especially after 38 weeks' gestation
- Hypoxia-induced peristalsis and sphincter relaxation
- Sequela to umbilical cord compression, which induces vagal stimulation in mature fetuses

Risk Factors

- Post-term dates
- Prolapsed cord
- Small for gestational age
- Fetal distress
- Intrauterine infection, such as chorioamnionitis or listeria vaginitis

Signs and Symptoms

- Green-tinged amniotic fluid
- A thick, fresh consistency of the meconium, passed in late labor is more likely to be a result of fetal distress.

Diagnostic Tests

Intervention is not done on the basis of meconium staining alone. The following tests are used to evaluate the need for interventions such as emergency cesarean birth:

- Fetal heart rate monitoring: presence of decreased variability, sinusoidal pattern Moderate-severe variable or late FHR decelerations, together with meconium staining, are an ominous sign.
- Fetal scalp blood sampling to check for acidosis

Therapeutic Nursing Management

- Closely monitor FHR.
- Monitor newborn's respiratory efforts carefully. Prevent aspiration of meconium by suctioning the upper respiratory tract immediately after birth (some suctioning at the perineum may be done as the head is delivered).
- Set up oxygen delivery apparatus (oxygen mask for blow by O_2 or mask continuous positive airway pressure).
- Administer oxygen as needed. The infant's color, perfusion, or signs of respiratory distress, such grunting, flaring, retractions, or apnea indicate that the infant requires supplementary oxygen.
- Prepare intubation equipment for deep endotracheal suctioning: endotracheal tube, laryngoscope, suctioning equipment, stylet (elective), and meconium aspirator (a DeLee apparatus may be used as an alternative). The nurse may assist with the procedure for cord visualization and/or endotracheal suctioning. Positioning of the infant is supine with the airway in a neutral position. Oxygen blow-by, bag-mask CPAP, or positive pressure ventilation may be necessary after the procedure. The infant will require stabilization of the extremities during the procedure.
- Be prepared to care for stressed infant. Transfer to newborn intensive care unit if condition deteriorates.

Complications (in the Newborn)

Fetal/newborn: Aspiration of meconium, pneumothorax, pneumonitis, aspiration pneumonia, persistent pulmonary hypertension (PPHN), asphyxia, seizures, renal failure, and death

Critical Thinking Exercise: Nursing Management of the Client with Meconium-Stained Amniotic Fluid

Situation: P.K. is 20 years old. She is gravida 1 para 0, and at 41 weeks gestation. She is in active first-stage labor. Her cervix is dilated to 6 cm. Her uterine contractions are strong; frequency is every 5 minutes, duration is 70 seconds. The FHR is 120 with decreased variability and frequent variable decelerations. The decision is made to apply a fetal scalp electrode in order to better evaluate the FHR. When the amniotomy is performed, about 750 mL of green-tinged fluid with small white particles is obtained.

1. What information should the nurse include when charting this event?

2. In preparation for this birth, the nurse should follow Neonatal Resuscitation principles. List five pieces of equipment that should be checked and ready for this baby's birth:

3. At the time of birth, the decisions regarding care are determined by the conditon of the baby and whether he/she is vigorous. What is included in this definition?

4. Describe the nursing care if the baby is vigorous at birth.

5. Describe the nursing care if the baby is not vigorous at birth.

Nursing Management of the Client with Labor Induction

Key Points

- Nursing care is similar for both augmentation and induction.
- Oxytocin can cause hyperstimulation and rupture of the uterus.
- For safety, oxytocin must be administered by infusion pump, never by gravity.
- Nursing care focuses on (a) monitoring labor progress, (b) monitoring FHR, and (c) observing for complications of oxytocin administration.
- If contractions are <2 min. apart, last longer than 90 seconds, or if the uterus does not relax completely between contractions: (a) stop the oxytocin, (b) administer oxygen, (c) place the woman in side-lying position, and (d) notify the primary care provider (follow same steps if fetal distress occurs).
- If the cervix is not favorable for induction, intravaginal prostaglandin gel may be used to soften the cervix prior to induction.
- **Key Terms/Concepts**: Induction, augmentation, amniotomy, oxytocic, laminaria

Overview

Induction of labor is the stimulation of the uterus to cause contractions before the spontaneous onset of labor. Augmentation of labor is the stimulation of uterine contractions after labor has started but is not progressing satisfactorily (e.g., as in hypotonic dysfunctional labor or dystocia). Stimulation of labor is most commonly achieved by: amniotomy (rupture of the membranes with an Amnihook or other sharp instrument), prostaglandin gel or laminaria for cervical ripening, and/or infusion of intravenous oxytocin (Pitocin, Syntocinon), which initiates or intensifies uterine contractions.

Some Indicators for Induction

- **Maternal indications**: Chorioamnionitis; chronic hypertension; insulin-dependent diabetes; pregnancy-induced hypertension (PIH); premature, preterm or prolonged rupture of membranes (PPPROM); or post-mature pregnancy.
- **Fetal indications**: Fetal demise, low biophysical profile, intrauterine growth retardation (IUGR), potential fetal jeopardy, post-term gestation, maternal-fetal blood incompatibility, oligohydramnios

Diagnostic Tests

- **Contraction stress test**: To assess fetal well-being
- **Gestational age assessment** via ultrasound or amniotomy
- Assessment of **fetal lung maturity** (L:S ratio)

- **Bishop score**: Assesses that cervix is soft, anterior, 50% effaced, and dilated 2 cm or more; and that the presenting part is engaged
- **Cervical exam** for "ripening"

Therapeutic Nursing Management

For amniotomy:

- Assess fetal heart rate before and immediately after procedure to detect cord compression or prolapse.
- Assess and record: time of rupture, color, odor, and consistency of the fluid.
- Monitor maternal temperature every two hours to rule out infection.
- Assess for signs of infection, such as maternal chills, fetal tachycardia, uterine tenderness, and foul-smelling vaginal drainage.
- Use comfort measures (e.g., cleanse perineum, change underpad frequently).
- Make careful observations for labor pattern changes.
- Assess maternal vital signs and urine output.
- Assess FHR frequently.

For oxytocin administration:

- Monitor FHR for 20 minutes before induction to establish fetal baseline status.
- Administer oxytocin via a secondary line (piggyback) so that it can be stopped in an emergency without discontinuing the primary/maintenance fluid.
- Increase dosage gradually, according to protocols, until an adequate contraction pattern is established. Dosage varies among individuals.
- Within the medical orders or institution protocols, the nurse decides when to start, change, or stop the oxytocin infusion.
- Monitor blood pressure and pulse frequently.
- Monitor intake and output to assess for fluid retention.
- Monitor for signs of water intoxication: headache, blurred vision, increased BP and respirations, rales, wheezing, and coughing.
- Monitor for uterine hyperstimulation (contractions lasting more than 90 seconds and occurring more frequently than every two minutes) and a uterine resting tone of >20 mmHg.
- Continuously monitor FHR for signs of fetal distress (bradycardia; tachycardia; absent variability; repeated, late, or prolonged decelerations).

EMERGENCY MEASURES for uterine hyperstimulation or nonreassuring FHR pattern:

- Turn off oxytocin infusion; increase rate of maintenance intravenous fluids.
- Administer oxygen by face mask per protocol or order.
- Position woman in side-lying position.
- Notify primary health care provider.

Pharmacologic Management

Oxytocin (Pitocin, Syntocinon)—A pituitary hormone that stimulates uterine contractions. Oxytocin is capable of producing strong uterine contractions in a short time even at minimal dosages. It is administered intravenously ("piggybacked" to a primary bag), by pump, in incremental doses until an effective contraction pattern is achieved. Hyperstimulation and other side effects appear to be dose related.

Prostaglandin E gel/suppository (Prepidil, Cervidil, Prostin)—Prostaglandins may be placed in the vagina to induce labor; however, they are not widely used for this purpose. More commonly, they are administered intravaginally before labor induction to soften and thin the cervix (oxytocin does not achieve this effect). The woman should lie flat for 15-20 minutes after gel insertion to prevent leakage. Adverse effects include hypertonic uterine contractions.

Laminaria: Hydrophilic (moisture-attracting) inserts. They are placed in the cervix, where they absorb water, swell, and gradually dilate the cervix mechanically.

Complications

- **Maternal:** Uterine rupture, amniotic fluid embolus, precipitous labor/delivery, cervical laceration, postpartum hemorrhage, water intoxication
- **Fetal:** Fetal distress

Critical Thinking Exercise: Nursing Management of the Client with Labor Induction

Situation: C. L. is having labor augmented with oxytocin. Her cervix is 5 cm dilated and fully effaced and her membranes have ruptured. She is being continuously monitored for uterine activity and fetal heart rate.

1. What safety measures should the nurse take when setting up and administering the oxytocin? Explain the rationale for each.

2. The monitor shows that C. L.'s contractions are now every three minutes lasting 90 seconds with no relaxation of the uterus between contractions.. What should the nurse do first?

3. Match the letters of the information in the left column with the correct medication. Some letters may be used for more than one medication.

_____ Laminaria	a. Stimulates contractions of uterine smooth muscle
_____ Prostaglandin E gel/suppository	b. Softens the cervix
_____ Oxytocin (Pitocin)	c. Dilates the cervix mechanically
	d. Can cause uterine hyperstimulation
	e. Administered intravenously via infusion pump

Situation: A woman is to have her labor induced at 39 weeks gestation. However, a Bishop score indicates that her cervix is not "ripe." Therefore, she is to have prostaglandin gel inserted intravaginally prior to the induction. She asks the nurse, "Why are you putting that stuff in me? Do I have a vaginal infection?"

4. How should the nurse respond?

Case Study: The Client in First Stage Labor

Situation: A 30-year-old client, G1 P0, is in labor. Her cervix is dilated 4-5 cm and 75% effaced. Her membranes are currently intact. She has received routine prenatal care and her pregnancy has been uncomplicated.

Primary care provider's orders include:

- NPO with ice chips
- IV D5NS at 100 cc/hour
- Demerol 50 mg intramuscular for pain
- Continuous external fetal monitoring

Assessment findings reveal:

- Client is discouraged, tired, diaphoretic and restless.
- She is complaining of pain and is asking about options for pain relief medication.

Instructions: Prioritize **four** nursing interventions as you provide care for the client. Write the number in the box to indicate the order of your interventions (#1 = first, #2 = second, etc.) and briefly state your rationale for each intervention.

INTERVENTIONS	PRIORITY	RATIONALE
Promote relaxation.		
Provide comfort measures, including pain relief, as ordered.		
Provide strategies for coping in 2nd stage labor.		
Increase contact time with client.		

About 45 minutes later, after pain medication has been administered, assessment data reveals:

- Contractions every 2-3 minutes lasting 60-90 seconds
- The client is complaining of nausea.
- States she, "Can't go on with this."
- Membranes ruptured

Interactive activity: With a partner, select the client concerns of highest priority and list the nursing interventions you would perform to meet client needs at this time.

CLIENT CONCERNS	NURSING INTERVENTION

Physiological Changes

Key Points

- It takes about six weeks for a woman's body to return to its pre-pregnant state.
- Enormous physiological adjustments are made during the puerperium.
- After an initial rise in the abdomen, the uterine fundus descends 1-2 cm/24 hours; it should not be palpable after the 9th postpartum day.
- The fundus must remain firm to prevent excessive bleeding from the placental site.
- If the fundus is higher than normal and displaced to the right, suspect a full bladder (which can cause uterine atony and excessive bleeding).
- The breasts begin secreting colostrum during pregnancy and begin producing milk 2-3 days after birth of the baby.
- Diuresis and diaphoresis are normal and common.
- Ongoing assessments include: vital signs, lochia, fundal height and firmness, bowel and bladder function, perineal healing, breasts, teaching needs, and comfort level.
- For episiotomy pain, give mild oral analgesics (e.g., acetaminophen with codeine); for afterpains, give nonsteroidal anti-inflammatory drugs (e.g., ibuprofen).
- The most serious complications are: postpartum hemorrhage, mastitis, and urinary tract infection, puerperal infection, and thrombophlebitis.
- **Key Terms/Concepts**: Puerperium, afterpains, diaphoresis, diuresis, fundus, involution, lochia rubra, lochia serosa, lochia alibi, breast engorgement, mastitis

Overview

The postpartum period (also referred to as the puerperium, or fourth trimester of pregnancy) is the interval between the birth of the baby and the return of the client's reproductive system to its non-pregnant state. It lasts approximately six weeks. During this time, the physiologic changes that occurred in pregnancy are reversed, so the mother's body again undergoes enormous change at the same time that she is making psychologic adjustments and incorporating a new member into the family. The mother's response to her infant during this time is influenced by many factors, including her energy level and comfort, the condition of the baby, existing family dynamics, and the care and support provided by health professionals.

Postpartum Changes

Reproductive System

- Within 12 hours after the birth, the uterine fundus may be palpated as high as 1 cm above the umbilicus. During the next few days, it descends 1-2 cm every 24 hours; it should not be palpable abdominally after the ninth postpartum day.

Maternal Newborn Nursing

- A firm, contracted uterus prevents excessive bleeding from the placental site. This is caused by uterine contractions that constrict and occlude underlying blood vessels at the placental site. Another result of the contractions is uterine involution, the process in which the uterus is reduced in size after delivery to the prepregnant size.

- Cervical os closes. Cervical edema may remain for two to three months.

- Normal estrogen levels return by 10 weeks.

- Ovulation occurs in 10 to 12 weeks for non-lactating women and 12 to 16 weeks for lactating women.

- **Afterpains** (uterine contractions) occur with varying intensity, especially with breastfeeding. Afterpains are usually more intense in multigravidas.

- Lochia occurs in three stages: **lochia rubra** (bright red) lasts for the first three days; **lochia serosa** (pinkish, watery) is present on days three to 10; and **lochia alba** (whitish tan) appears after the 10th day (sometimes as late as six weeks).

Breasts

- Colostrum is secreted immediately after delivery.

- Milk production begins two to three days after delivery.

- Engorgement may occur.

Cardiovascular System

- Blood volume decreases after day three, as the excess fluid accumulated in pregnancy is eliminated. **Diaphoresis** eliminates much of the fluid via the skin, and heavy perspiration is normal for the first few days.

- Cardiac output and stroke volume decrease after the third week.

- Hemodilution immediately after delivery is followed by increased hematocrit for three to seven days. Hematocrit returns to normal by four to five weeks.

- White blood cell count is elevated for the first 12 days, and then returns to normal by the second week.

- Clotting factors remain elevated in the immediate puerperium (contributing to an increased risk for thrombophlebitis), but return to normal by the third week.

Respiratory System

- Respiratory function (tidal volume) returns to non-pregnant state within six months.

Urinary System

- Diuresis, beginning within 12 hours after delivery, is another mechanism in the reversal of the water metabolism of pregnancy. Urinary output may be 3000 cc per day during the first week.

- Bladder tone is restored by the end of the first week.

- Normal renal functioning returns by six weeks.

- Edema of the perineum, including the urethra, may cause difficult voiding and urinary retention during the first 24 hours postpartum.

Gastrointestinal System

- Normal bowel function returns by the end of the first week. Stool softeners may be used if episiotomy is present.
- In the immediate puerperium, the woman may be very hungry and thirsty.

Vital Signs

- Vital signs do not change much under normal circumstances.
- Temperature may rise slightly during first 24 hours due to dehydration.
- Pulse elevated slightly for first hour after birth; decreases to prepregnant rate by eight to 10 weeks.
- Respiration rate decreases to normal prebirth range by six to eight weeks.
- Blood pressure usually not altered; orthostatic hypotension may occur during first 48 hours.

Care of the Postpartum Client

General principles or goals of postpartum care include:
- Prevent hemorrhage
- Promote comfort
- Promote bowel elimination
- Promote urinary elimination
- Promote successful infant feeding
- Promote rest and return to normal activity
- Promote adequate nutritional intake
- Promote psychological well-being
- Promote client safety

General considerations for postpartum nursing assessment include: evaluate prenatal and intrapartal history for risk factors, provide privacy and encourage client to void prior to assessment, position client in bed with head flat for most accurate findings, proceed in a head-to-toe direction, vital signs are more accurate with the client at rest and will determine the priority for other assessments.

Vital Sign assessment parameters specific to the postpartum client:
- Temperature
  - Above 100.4° F after first 24 hours may indicate an infection
  - May be elevated initially after delivery related to dehydration
- Pulse
  - Normal range postpartum is 50-80 beats per minute
  - Pulse greater than 100 bpm should be reported to the healthcare provider
- Respirations
  - Normal range is 16-24 breaths per minute
- Blood pressure
  - Assess for orthostatic hypotension
  - Monitor more closely if client has a history or preeclampsia

- Women who experience operative procedures, cesarean delivery, or tubal ligation have postpartal needs similar to those of women who gave birth vaginally and the needs of postoperative clients; monitor breath sounds and have the client cough and take deep breaths.

Preventing Hemorrhage

For the postpartum client, the nurse must:

- Assess for risk factors: Delivery of a large infant, multiple gestation, polyhydramnious, multiparity, precipitous delivery, dystocia, prolonged third stage, retained placental fragments, medication use (general anesthesia, tocolytics, magnesium sulfate therapy, low platelet count related to PIH)
- Keep bladder empty
- Gently massage fundus; if boggy, teach self-massage of fundus.
- Administer oxytocic medications if ordered: oxytocin (Pitocin), methylergonovine maleate (Methergine), ergonovine maleate (Ergonate)
- Monitor side effects of oxytocics, if administered:
  - Hypotension with rapid IV bolus of Pitocin
  - Hypertension with Methergine and Ergonate

Promote comfort:

- Provide warm blankets for "postpartum chill" (shivering due to work of labor and birth) during the first two hours.
- Apply ice to perineum 20 minutes on/and 10 minutes off for first 24 hours.
- Encourage sitz bath, warm or cool, tid and prn after first 12-24 hours.
- Teach client perineal care to be used after every elimination by pouring warm water over the perineum. Next, dry from front to back to prevent tissue trauma and contamination from the anal area. Then, apply clean perineal pad from front to back without touching the surface that will be next to client.
- Teach client to tighten buttocks, then sit and relax muscles.
- Apply topical anesthetics (Dermoplast or Americaine spray) or witch hazel compress (Tucks).
- Administer analgesics: acetaminophen, NSAIDs (ibuprofen), narcotics (codeine, hydrocodone, oxycodone).
- Utilize PCA or morphine epidural for cesarean deliveries.
- Monitor for side effects of morphine epidural, if administered; late-onset respiratory depression (eight to 12 hours), nausea and vomiting (four to seven hours), itching (within three and up to 10 hours), urinary retention, and somnolence.

Promote bowel elimination:

- Encourage frequent and early ambulation
- Encourage increased fluids and fiber
- Administer stool softeners as ordered: suppositories are contraindicated if the client has lacerations.

Promote bladder elimination:

- Encourage voiding or attempting to void every two to three hours.

- Foley catheter may be ordered for the first 12-24 after cesarean birth
- Catheterize for urinary retention as ordered.

Promote successful infant feeding patterns

- Suppression of lactation and bottle feeding
  - Utilize snug bra or breast binder continuously for five to seven days to prevent engorgement.
  - Avoid heat and stimulation to the breasts.
  - Apply ice packs for 20 minutes, qid, if engorgement occurs.
  - Encourage demand feedings every three to four hours, awakening during the day and allowing to sleep at night
- Establishment of lactation and successful breast feeding
  - Refer to Chapter 42

Promote rest and gradual return to activity

- Cluster nursing care to avoid frequent interruptions
- Plan rest periods for mother when the baby is expected to sleep.
- Teach the woman to resume activity gradually over four to five weeks; avoid lifting, stair climbing, and strenuous activity.
- Simple postpartal exercises should be started; encourage the client to strengthen muscles affected by childbearing.
- Increased lochia or pain indicates overexertion; modify exercise plan.

Promote adequate nutritional intake

- Encourage fluid intake of 2,000 mL per day.
- Encourage lactating mother's to increase diet by 500 Kcal/day.
- Instruct the client to continue her prenatal vitamins and iron as ordered. Instruct her that iron is better absorbed in the presence of vitamin C and that iron may increase constipation.

Promote psychological well-being

- Plan care based upon the client's phase of adjustment and degree of independence.
- Provide choices when possible.
- Encourage expression of feelings.
- Encourage the client to tell her birth story
- Provide recognition for the client's self-care and her infant care.

Promote client safety

- Administer RhoGam as indicated.
  - Confirm the woman is a candidate: Rh-negative mother not sensitized (negative indirect Coombs' test), Rh-positive newborn not sensitized (negative direct Coombs' test), and no known maternal allergy to globulin preparations.
  - Administer 300 ug IM within 72 hours of delivery.
- Administer rubella vaccination if indicated.
  - Refer to Chapter 15.

- Teach warning signs to report to primary care giver
  - Bright red bleeding saturating more than one pad per hour or passing large clots
  - Temperature greater than 100.4° F
  - Excessive pain
  - Chills
  - Reddened or warm areas of the breast
  - Reddening or gaping episiotomy, foul smelling lochia
  - Inability to urinate; burning, frequency, or urgency with urination
  - Calf pain, tenderness, redness, or swelling

Diagnostic Tests

- Hematocrit/hemoglobin
- CBC
- Antibody screen

Complications

- Postpartum hemorrhage (large amount of vaginal bleeding)
- Puerperal infection
  - Changes in lochia (e.g., amount, odor, change to earlier character)
  - Fever
  - Redness, drainage from episiotomy
  - Pain or tenderness in abdomen or pelvis
- Thrombophlebitis: localized pain, redness, swelling or warm spot in calf
- Mastitis: breast pain, redness, tenderness, swelling
- Urinary tract infection: pain/burning urination

Critical Thinking Exercise: Physiological Changes

Situation: C.J. gave birth to her baby at 8 a.m. The nurse's assessment findings at 8 p.m. are as follows: BP 120/80, pulse 70, respirations 16, temperature 99.5° F, uterine fundus 1 cm above the umbilicus and right of midline, breasts are soft. C.J. says she has been perspiring alot.

1. Which of the nurse's findings need to be explored further, that is, which findings could be an indication that a problem is developing?

2. What is probably causing C.J.'s slightly elevated temperature?

3. What other information does the nurse need in order to interpret the meaning of C.J.'s temperature reading?

4. What further data does the nurse need in order to adequately interpret the meaning of "fundus 1 cm above the umbilicus and right of midline"?

5. The nurse is caring for a client in the immediate postpartum period. While assessing for each of these potential complications after delivery, which clinical manifestations will the nurse most likely identify? Match the clinical findings with the complication.

____ Postpartum hemorrhage	a. Uterus boggy and high in abdomen
____ Puerperal infection	b. Foul-smelling lochia
____ Urinary tract infection	c. Temperature of 102° F
____ Thrombophlebitis	d. Large amount of lochia rubra, blood in the bed
	e. Burning with urination
	f. Quarter-sized red, warm area on calf
	g. Abdominal and pelvic pain
	h. Frequent urination
	i. Pain with dorsiflexion

Nursing Management/Teaching for the Client who is Breastfeeding

Key Points

- The breasts produce colostrum during pregnancy and immediately after birth of the baby; it is replaced by milk in two to four days after birth.
- Colostrum is nourishing for the baby; it also contains antibodies.
- The first two hours after birth are optimal for beginning breastfeeding (infant is in a quiet, alert state).
- To prevent sore nipples, teach the woman to: position the baby properly; assess for correct suck and swallow; avoid using soap on her nipples; avoid plastic-lined bras; release suction with her finger before removing baby from the breast;   and avoid prolonged periods of non-nutritive breastfeeding.
- Signs of mastitis include: redness (especially localized redness), swelling, tenderness of a breast (mastitis is usually unilateral), and fever.
- Cracked nipples are a portal of entry for pathogens and a risk factor for mastitis.
- Teach the client to wash hands prior to feedings.
- **Key Terms/Concepts**: Colostrum, transitional milk, afterpains, engorgement, mastitis

Overview

Breastfeeding provides the infant with nutrition via breast milk. The first two hours after birth are optimum for encouraging breastfeeding because the infant is in an alert state. Breastfeeding stimulates uterine contractions, helping to prevent maternal hemorrhage. Breast discomfort in the postpartum period is usually due to engorgement and dissipates in 24 to 48 hours.

Colostrum is the first secretion produced, beginning in late pregnancy and continuing for several days after birth. Colostrum is a thick, yellow, creamy fluid containing high levels of antibodies, protein, and fat-soluble vitamins that nourish the baby until milk is produced. In two to four days after birth, colostrum is replaced by transitional milk. Produced for about two weeks, transitional milk provides more calories and is higher in fat, lactose, and water-soluble vitamins. Mature milk is produced after about two weeks postpartum. It has higher water content and looks "thin" although it is nutritionally complete for the baby.

Therapeutic Nursing Management

- Instruct client that breasts must be kept clean and to wash breasts at the beginning of the shower each day. If breastfeeding, do not use soap on nipples.

- Air dry nipples following feedings to prevent excess moisture inside bra. Use disposable bra pads to absorb leaking milk; change frequently to prevent infection. Do not use pads with plastic liners.

- Use cold compresses or ice packs or place fresh cabbage leaves inside the bra between feedings to relieve engorgement discomfort. Heat and massage should be used just before feedings to increase milk flow. If the areola is too engorged for the infant to latch on, the mother should express milk by hand or with a breast pump.

- For mothers with engorgement, it may help to medicate them with a mild analgesic 15 to 30 minutes before feeding.

- Teach to wear well-fitting support bra or breast binder for the first 72 hours, even at night, for lactation suppression.

- Teach danger signs of postpartum breast complications:
  - Redness
  - Swelling
  - Fever
  - Tenderness
  - Cracked nipples

- Teach breast self-exam (performed monthly).

- Assist client to position infant and initiate early feedings (time of infant reactivity is best).

- Teach client to wash hands prior to feedings. The average time for feeding is 30 minutes, or approximately 15 minutes per breast. Infant should be put to breast every two to three hours for the first few days of life.

- Prevent sore nipples by varying infant positions during feeding:
  - Side-lying
  - Cradle (sitting)
  - Football hold

- Release suction (use finger) before removing baby from breast.

- Refer client to lactation consultant as appropriate.

Complications

- **Afterpains**: A common discomfort in multiparas when uterine involution occurs. Breastfeeding causes uterine contraction by stimulating release of oxytocin. Thus, the client who is breastfeeding may experience increased discomfort when the neonate nurses.

- Sore nipples

- Dehydration in infant; Poor skin turgor, lethargy, sunken fontanels, decreased urine, failure to thrive

- Mastitis/infection

Critical Thinking Exercise: Nursing Management/ Teaching for the Client who is Breastfeeding

Situation: A woman has just given birth to her first baby. She wishes to breastfeed her baby, but she has not been to any parent education classes. She says, "I don't even know how to begin."

1. Write a useful nursing diagnosis for this woman.

2. Write goals/expected outcomes for this nursing diagnosis.

3. The woman asks, "How long should I let the baby nurse on each breast?" What should the nurse tell her?

4. What should the nurse teach the woman about techniques preventing nipple trauma?

5. On the first postpartum day, the woman says, "I've heard that my milk won't come in for two or three days. Is there any point in letting the baby breastfeed now? Will the baby even get anything?" What should the nurse tell her?

Situation: Ms. R., a recent immigrant from India, has given birth to her first child. She wishes to breastfeed but states that her mother has advised her that colostrum is harmful to the baby. She wishes to begin breastfeeding when her "milk comes in" around the third day.

6. What information does Ms. R. need in order to make an informed choice regarding infant nutrition?

7. What options might you explore with her?

8. What follow-up would be important to her decision to breastfeed?

Bonding

Key Points

- Bonding is facilitated by parent-infant contact during the first hour after birth.
- Attachment can still occur even if parent-infant contact is not possible during this sensitive period (e.g., in the event of a medical emergency).
- Bonding behaviors include en face position, calling baby by name (instead of "it" or "he"), identifying baby's unique characteristics and relating them to other family members, and holding the infant close to the body.
- Promote bonding/attachment by delaying procedures during the first hour after birth in order to provide unlimited parent-infant contact.
- Promote bonding by role modeling attachment behaviors and pointing out the infant's responses to verbal stimulation.
- **Key Terms/Concepts**: Bonding, attachment, en face position, sensitive period, bonding behaviors

Overview

The process by which a parent and child come to love and accept each other is called attachment or bonding. Attachment begins during pregnancy and intensifies during the early postpartum period. It is developed and maintained by contact and interaction with the infant. With today's family-centered care, nurses try to adapt childbirth in an effort to promote bonding and integration of the infant into the family unit. Bonding is enhanced by parent-infant interaction during the sensitive period that occurs during the first hours following birth. The infant is in a quiet, alert stage during this time, with the eyes open so that he/she seems to gaze directly at the parent(s). The infant will respond to voice and touch at this time.

Factors Affecting Bonding

- Mother's emotional and physical condition after labor
- Infant's condition and behavior
- Separation of mother and infant after birth due to maternal or infant illness
- Desparity between fantasy and reality related to birthing experience and new role as a mother
- Maternal drug or alcohol abuse
- Neonatal congenital anomalies
- Prematurity

- Teenage mother
- Unwanted pregnancy
- Infant is the product of rape or incest

Parental Behaviors Indicating that Bonding is Occurring

- En face position, eye contact
- Calls infant by name
- Assigns meanings to infant's actions
- Talks to, coos, or sings to infant
- Touches: progressing from fingertip to fingers to palms to holding close (full body contact)
- Claims infant as family member

Parental Behaviors Indicating Bonding Problems

- Ignoring infant's presence
- Turning away from infant
- Wakes baby when sleeping; handles roughly
- Expresses disappointment, displeasure in infant
- Disgusted by infant's body fluids (e.g., urine, spit-up)
- Apathy in participating in newborn's care

Therapeutic Nursing Management

- Help parent(s) to identify baby's unique characteristics.
- Encourage family to hold, cuddle, inspect, and feed the newborn.
- Point out normal newborn reflexes and abilities.
- Place infant skin-to-skin with mother soon after birth.
- Provide privacy and an environment that enhances family-infant interaction.

Complications

- Failure to thrive/neglect
- Non-attachment/physical abuse
- Emotional detachment

Critical Thinking Exercise: Bonding

Situation: A 16-year-old gave birth to a baby boy three hours ago. It was a vaginal birth and she has a midline episiotomy and hemorrhoids. She asks the nurse to take her baby to the nursery for a few hours, saying, "Please take care of it for a while. I am exhausted. I was in labor for 16 hours and had no sleep at all last night. I really need to sleep." The baby is lying across the mother's lap and the mother does not u   nfold the baby before handing him to the nurse.

1. What signs (defining characteristics) of delayed bonding is the mother exhibiting?

2. What risk factors are present that should alert the nurse to the possibility of delayed bonding?

3. Is there enough data to infer that there is an attachment/bonding problem?

4. What would be an appropriate nursing diagnosis for this situation?

5. Prioritize the mother's needs at this time. Explain your thinking.

_____Sleep and rest

_____Interaction time with the baby to facilitate bonding

_____Learn how to hold and cuddle the baby

6 What are the important nursing interventions for this woman at this time? Explain your thinking.

7. After the mother is rested, what other physical condition will the nurse need to assess to be sure that it is not interfering with the mother's ability to bond?

Situation: A 16-year-old gave birth to a male infant six hours ago. You are the nurse providing care to this new mother and her infant. The mother and infant's vital signs are stable. You bring the portable bathtub to the bedside for the baby's first bath after discussion with the teenage mother. She is tired but eager to learn how to care for her infant.

8. Describe eight things that could be incorporated in this interactive bathing opportunity.

Nursing Management of the Client with Postpartum Hemorrhage and Disseminated Intravascular Coagulation (DIC)

Key Points

- PPH is excessive blood loss after childbirth.
- The most frequent cause of PPH is uterine atony.
- Predisposing factors for uterine atony are:
  - Overdistension of the uterus from any cause
  - Uterine fatigue (e.g., from prolonged labor)
  - Bladder distention
- Prevent/treat uterine atony by:
  - Being aware of risk factors
  - Inducing voiding to prevent bladder distention
  - Massaging the uterine fundus if it is not firm
- Assess for signs of hemorrhage: heavy lochia, and boggy uterus.
- The most serious complication is hypovolemic shock.
- If PPH occurs, massage fundus, notify birth attendant, administer oxytocics as ordered, and be aware that a D & C may be necessary.
- **Key Terms/Concepts**: Early postpartum hemorrhage (PPH), delayed PPH, hypovolemic shock, fundal massage, coagulopathy, uterine atony, clotting mechanisms, purpura, petechiae, ecchymoses, fibrinogen

Overview

Postpartum hemorrhage (PPH) is the loss of more than 500 mL of blood after vaginal childbirth, or 1000 mL after cesarean birth. The most common cause of PPH is uterine atony, which complicates about one in 20 births. Less frequent causes are retained placenta, lacerations, and coagulopathies. Any excessive bleeding should be treated as hemorrhage during the postpartum period. Initial treatment of suspected postpartum hemorrhage is by prompt fundal massage and notification of the birth attendant.

Early, or immediate, PPH develops within 24 hours of birth. Late PPH usually occurs after the woman returns home. It is usually caused by subinvolution of the uterus, retained placental fragments, or infection.

Risk Factors

- Uterine muscle overstretched or fatigued (e.g., by large infant, multiple births, long labor, precipitous labor, multiparity)
- Retained placenta
- Subinvolution of the uterus

- Vaginal laceration
- Hematoma
- Muscle relaxation/drugs
- PIH (Pregnancy-induced hypertension)
- Distended bladder
- Inverted uterus
- Oxytocin induction or augmentation of labor

Signs and Symptoms

- Increased bloody lochia—can be constant trickle, steady flow, or large gush of bright red blood and clots from the vagina
- Saturation of more than one peripad per hour
- Severe, unrelieved rectal or perineal pain (signs of hematoma)
- Soft or "boggy" uterus (may be enlarged)
- Tachycardia, hypotension, decreased urinary output (signs of hypovolemic shock)

Diagnostic Tests

- Hematocrit
- Hemoglobin

Therapeutic Nursing Management

- Continually assess for signs of shock.
- Insert indwelling catheter with urometer.
- Monitor for urinary output of at least 30 mL/hr.
- Palpate uterus frequently for consistency, location, and size.
- Check lochia for color, amount, and large clots.
- Inspect perineum for lacerations, hematoma, or disrupted episiotomy.
- Monitor urine output/bladder distention.
- Monitor vital signs, level of consciousness, and skin color/warmth.
- Question excessive pain.
- Massage uterus and administer oxytocics as ordered. (Oxytocics are administered to expel retained placental fragments and to contract an atonic uterus).
- Notify birth attendant if vital signs are abnormal or if complications arise.
- Prepare client for D & C (dilatation and curettage) if manual removal of placental fragments is required.
- Support client and family.
- Administer oxygen and medications as ordered.
- Insert a straight catheter to empty distended bladder.

Nursing Treatment to Prevent Postpartum Hemorrhage

- Inspect placenta for missing parts.
- Administer oxytocics.
- Maintain open IV line.
- Apply ice to the perineum.
- Induce voiding; insert a straight catheter to empty distended bladder.
- Massage fundus if boggy.
- Monitor lochia amount and type.
- On discharge, teach client to report:
  - The return of bright red lochia after 4th postpartum day
  - Signs of infection, which may cause delayed postpartum hemorrhage:
    - Fever over 100.4° F
    - Foul-smelling lochia
    - Flu-like symptoms

Pharmacologic Management

- Intravenous infusion of 20 units of oxytocin in 1,000 mL of lactated Ringer's or normal saline solution
- Ergonovine (Ergotrate) or methylergonovine (Methergine)— intramuscularly (IM) or intravenously
- Prostaglandin F (carboprost tromethamine)— intramuscular or intramyometrially

Complications

- Hypovolemic shock
- Occult bleeding: blood stays within the uterus, distending it. It is difficult to recognize. On palpation, uterus is soft, boggy, and enlarged.
- Postpartum hemorrhage can be life-threatening. Uncorrected blood loss results in loss of consciousness, renal failure, and death.
- Retained placenta can cause uterine infection, subinvolution, and subsequent hemorrhage.

Disseminated Intravascular Coagulation (DIC)

Overview

DIC is among the most common blood clotting disorders that occur after delivery to postpartum clients where there is an acceleration of the clotting mechanism and activation of the fibrinogen system. This occurs as a complication of severe postpartum hemorrhage (as from an abruption), infection, retained dead fetus, amniotic fluid embolism.

Other conditions that may precipate DIC

- Shock
- Cirrhosis
- Glomerulonephritis
- Acute fulminate hepatitis
- Acute bacterial and viral infections
- Conditions that may cause release of platelet factor II
    - Fat emboli, snake bites
    - Hemolytic processes due to infection, transfusion reactions, immunologic disorders
    - Tissue damage due to trauma, heat stroke, extensive burns, transplant, surgery
- Conditions that may cause release of thromboplastin from the tissues
    - Neoplastic growths
    - Obstetric conditions mentioned earlier

DIC Pathophysiology

- Disease state
- Release of thomboplastic substances
- Activation of fibrinogen
- Deposition of fibrin throughout microcirculation
- Platelet aggregation increases causing clot formation in the brain, kidneys, ear, and other organs.
- Hemolysis of trapped RBCs causes sluggishness circulation and cellular hypoxia, and lack of nutrients.
- Platelets, prothrombin, other clotting factors consumed in the process
- Excessive clotting activates fibrolytic mechanism, causing production of fibrin split products.
- Fibrin split products inhibit platelet clotting --> leading to further bleeding
- With clots being formed and clotting factors depleted, the blood loses its ability to clot.

Clinical Manifestations

Onset is usually acute and develops within days to hours after the initial assault to the body system.

- Subacute DIC may not be apparent initially but may fulminate as the clinical course progresses.
- Chronic DIC may develop in cases of clients with cancer or women carrying a dead fetus.
- Manifestations may be mild or extremely severe in nature.

Signs and Symptoms

- Purpura, petechiae, and ecchymoses on the skin, mucous membranes, heart lining, and lungs
- Prolonged bleeding from a venipuncture
- Severe uncontrolled hemorrage during surgery or childbirth
- Oliguria and acute renal failure
- Convulsions and coma, which may terminate in death

Laboratory Tests

Lab findings in severe cases indicate that the hemostatic system has totally failed

Test	Results
Prothrombin time	Prolonged
Partial prothrombin time	Usually prolonged
Thrombin time	Usually prolonged
Fibrinogen level	Usually depressed
Platelet count	Usually depressed
Fibrin split products	Elevated
Protamine sulfate test	Strongly positive
Factor assays II, V, VII	Reduced

Nursing Management of the Client with DIC

- Prevention
- Reverse the pathological clotting.
- Control bleeding and shock.
- Detect occult bleeding.
- Prevent further bleeding.
- Accurately determine blood loss.
- Administer blood products and meds as prescribed.
- Observe for and report transfusion reactions and medication side affects.
- Assess all body systems for effects of DIC.
- Nursing care depends on the severity of the process:
  - General goal is to monitor and quantify blood loss and provide supportive therapy and blood components.

- Monitor laboratory test to determine effectiveness of treatment.
- Observe for signs of thrombosis.
- Avoid further complications.
- Avoid infections.
- Apply pressure to bleeding sites.
- Turn and reposition frequently and gently.
- This condition results in overt bleeding from body orifices and other clinical symptoms are frightening.
- Offer strong emotional support.

Critical Thinking Exercise: Nursing Management of the Client with Postpartum Hemorrhage and Disseminated Intravascular Coagulation (DIC)

Situation: N.C., a 35-year-old multipara gave birth to a 9 lb. 14 oz. baby two hours ago after a rapid labor. She has saturated three peripads since the birth. Her fundus is firm and at the level of the umbilicus. Her vital signs are within normal limits.

1. Which data should alert the nurse that N.C. is at risk for postpartum hemorrhage?

2. The risk factors for postpartum hemorrhage have been described as the four Ts. What are they?

3. At the next assessment, the nurse determines that N.C.'s fundus is soft. Other data are unchanged. What are the priority interventions? Explain your reasoning.

4. After the nurse performs the interventions in #3, N.C. continues to bleed heavily. The nurse notifies the primary care provider, administers 20 units of oxytocin through her IV line according to protocols, and continues to monitor the bleeding. What are the most important vital signs to monitor at this time? Why?

5. The nurse also implements a medical order to insert an indwelling urinary catheter. What is the rationale for doing this?

Case Study: The Client Diagnosed with Postpartum Hemorrhage

Situation: Six hours ago, a 29-year-old client (gravida 3, para 3) vaginally gave birth to a male infant. About two hours after delivery, the client began to bleed steadily and the estimated blood loss currently is about 700 mL. Thus far, the client has received one unit of blood and presently is receiving IV fluids at 150 cc per hour. She has a Foley catheter in place. Vital signs at 2 pm are: BP 100/60, P 100, and R 12. Hematocrit is 24%. You are assigned to care for the client on the postpartum unit during the evening shift.

Instructions: Prioritize the nursing interventions you would perform when providing care for the client. Write the number in the box to identify the order of your interventions (#1 = first, #2 = second, etc.)

INTERVENTIONS	PRIORITY #
Assess uterus for consistency, firmness, and position.	
Monitor urine output. Assess accurately intake and output.	
Note amount and character of lochia.	
Assess breath sounds.	
Take vital signs.	
Review lab values.	
Explain plan of care to woman/family	

The client has laboratory work done on your shift and a repeat hematocrit at eight hours post-delivery is 29%. She receives another unit of blood.

Instructions: Based on the lab data, identify the priority problem and the nursing interventions for this situation.

PROBLEM

1.

2.

NURSING INTERVENTIONS

Which information would indicate that the client's condition is improving?

Three days after birth the client's hematocrit is 33% and she is not experiencing any abnormal bleeding. She is planning to be discharged the next day.

Instructions: Work with a partner to develop a discharge-teaching plan for the client.

Nursing Management of the Client with Postpartum Infection

Key Points

- General symptoms include: Fever >100.4° F (38° C) after the first 24 hours and lasting two or more successive days; chills, flu-like symptoms, elevated WBCs and, uterine subinvolution.
- Other symptoms vary according to the site of the infection.
- The most common postpartum infections are: reproductive tract infection, wound infection, urinary tract infection, and mastitis.
- Complications are sepsis, peritonitis, and paralytic ileus.
- Nursing care involves administration of antibiotics and relieving pain.
- **Key terms**: Puerperal infection, mastitis, metritis, sepsis, uterine involution

Overview

Puerperal infection is any infection of the reproductive tract that occurs within 28 days after abortion or childbirth. The first symptom is usually a fever. Common sources of postpartum infection are endometritis, mastitis, episiotomy or incision infection, urinary tract infections, and respiratory infections. Metritis is an infection of the uterus that usually begins as an infection at the placental site. It is the most common postpartum infection.

Risk Factors

- Highly vascular uterine lining and raw placental implant site
- Prolonged labor
- Diabetes mellitus
- Substance abuse
- Malnutrition
- Prolonged, preterm, rupture of membranes (PPROM)
- Cesarean birth
- Manual extraction of the placenta
- Retained placental fragments
- Anemia
- Obesity
- Hematomas
- Epidural anesthesia
- Chorioamnionitis
- Contact with an infectious agent

Signs and Symptoms

- Fever higher than 100.4° F (38° C) after the first 24 hours that lasts two or more successive days
- Chills
- Tachycardia
- Uterine subinvolution
- Elevated white blood cell count
- Flu-like symptoms: fever, chills, nausea and vomiting, anorexia, fatigue, headache
- Reproductive tract infection: backache, abdominal pain/tenderness, foul smelling lochia, purulent discharge
- Wound infection: erythema, warmth, swelling, tenderness, edges not approximated, purulent drainage
- Urinary tract infection: pain, burning, urgency, or frequency of urination
- Mastitis: Pain, erythema, or warmth in the breast along with flu-like symptoms

Diagnostic Tests and Labs

- Vaginal examination and lochial cultures
- CBC (However, leukocytes are normally as high as 20,000-30,000 for a short time after labor and birth.)

Therapeutic Nursing Management

- Evaluate vital signs each shift.
- Inspect perineum or cesarean incision.
- Assess lochia.
- Assess uterine involution.
- Attend to complaint of pain, dysuria, nausea/vomiting, or diarrhea.
- Assist client with warm sitz baths to promote healing in mild cases of local infection.
- Ensure adequate fluid and nutritional intake.
- Comfort measures include warm blankets for chilling, cool compresses, sponge baths, perineal care, and a heating pad.
- Obtain specimens per order or protocols (e.g., urine, blood, culture from cervix).
- Monitor response to antibiotics—clinical signs usually improve within 48 to 72 hours.
- The client with metritis should be placed in Fowler's position to promote drainage of lochia.
- Instruct the client in handwashing techniques.
- Teach the mother to watch for thrush in the infant (white patches on tongue and buccal mucosa).

Pharmacologic Management

- Administer acetaminophen (Tylenol) or topical sprays for pain relief in local infections.
- Administer intravenous antibiotics if ordered.

Complications

- Sepsis, septic shock
- Peritonitis
- Paralytic ileus

Critical Thinking Exercise: Nursing Management of the Client with Postpartum Infection

Situation: An obese woman is admitted to the postpartum unit after a cesarean birth. The cesarean was performed for fetal distress after a 16-hour labor. Her history includes two prior miscarriages and prolonged rupture of membranes before this birth. Two days after the birth, the nurse observes that the edges of her abdominal incision are not approximated; the skin around the incision is red and the wound is draining a small amount of seropurulent drainage. The wound is painful and tender to touch.

1. What risk factors for infection are present?

2. What symptoms of infection are present?

3. What other assessments should the nurse make that are related to puerperal infection?

4. What interventions will be initiated by the nurse?

5. What other orders would be appropriate for this patient?

Nursing Management of the Client with Mastitis

Key Points

- Mastitis usually occurs during the second and third weeks after birth, although it may develop at any time during breastfeeding.
- Mastitis usually affects only one breast.
- Localized signs/symptoms: area of redness and inflammation on the breast, enlarged, tender auxiliary lymph nodes.
- Generalized signs/symptoms: Fever of 101.1° F or higher, chills, malaise, headache, and aching muscles.
- Nursing measures focus on promoting comfort and maintaining lactation.
- **Key Terms/Concepts**: Staph aureus, unilateral infection, client teaching, hygenic practices

Overview

Mastitis is an infection of the breast in the postpartum period. The organism is usually hemolytic Staphylococcal aureus. The initial lesion is usually an infected nipple fissure. Inflammation and edema cause engorgement and obstruction of milk flow. Mastitis occurs two to four weeks after delivery and generally affects just one side. It is most common in first-time mothers who are breastfeeding. Most cases of acute mastitis can be avoided by careful hand washing and proper breastfeeding technique, which prevents cracked nipples.

Risk Factors

- Sore/cracked nipples
- Poor maternal hygiene
- Poor positioning of the nipple in infant's mouth
- Excessive or vigorous infant sucking
- Decreased breastfeeding due to supplemental bottles
- Fatigue, stress, other health problems that may decrease resistance to micro-organisms
- Maternal dehydration

Signs and Symptoms

- Local pain, erythema, heat in breast
- Flu-like symptoms: fever, chills, malaise, body aches, headache
- Axillary adenopathy

Diagnostic Tests and Lab

- CBC
- Cultures of drainage

Therapeutic Nursing Management

- Assess breastfeeding practices.
- Prevention: Teach mother proper breastfeeding technique, positioning of the baby, how to prepare her nipples for breastfeeding, and care of her breasts postpartum.
- Teach mother the signs of mastitis before discharge.
- Apply warm compresses and encourage frequent feeding on affected side.
- Encourage rest, fluids, and analgesics to promote comfort.
- Administer antibiotics as prescribed.
- Reassure mother she is not exposing her newborn to infection.
- Counsel mother to continue breastfeeding. Lactation can be maintained by breastfeeding, manual expression, or pumping the breasts every two to four hours to empty them.
- Teach the mother to empty the breast completely at each feeding to prevent stasis of milk, which can result in an abscess.
- Encourage a fluid intake of at least 3,000 mL per day.

Pharmacology

- Antibiotics (cephalosporins and vancomycin)

Complications

- Inhibition of letdown reflex due to maternal discomfort
- Breast abscess

Critical Thinking Exercise: Nursing Management of the Client with Mastitis

Situation: Two weeks after giving birth, a woman calls the care provider's office because, she says, "Something is wrong with my breast." Upon further questioning, she says that she has a hot, hard, sore spot "about the size of a golfball" on her left breast. She says that she has been having chills and a headache.

1. What advice will be given to this woman?

2. What symptoms would lead the nurse to suspect mastitis instead of breast engorgement?

3. The woman says, "I think I may have an infection, so I've been bottle-feeding my baby so she won't get sick." What should the nurse tell her?

4. What other advice should the nurse provide regarding follow-up, infant nutrition, and self care?

Nursing Management of the Client with Thrombophlebitis

| Key Points |

- Prevention—early ambulation and adequate hydration
- Assessment: Monitor status of the thrombosis (e.g., measure leg circumference of each leg and compare results), degree of pain, and symptoms of pulmonary embolism.
- Treatment may include anticoagulant therapy, bedrest, and elevation of the leg, elastic support stockings, and warm packs to the leg.
- For clients receiving heparin, monitor laboratory reports and observe for signs of bleeding.
- Protamine sulfate is the antidote for heparin; vitamin K is the antidote for warfarin.
- **Key Terms/Concepts**: Thrombus, thrombophlebitis, superficial thrombus, deep vein thrombus, pulmonary embolus, inflammation, hypercoagulability, stasis

Overview

Thrombophlebitis is inflammation of a vessel wall in association with a thrombus. A thrombus is the formation of a blood clot inside a blood vessel that is caused by injury or inflammation of the vessel wall, reduced velocity of blood flow (venous stasis), and hypercoagulability of the blood. Two causes of thrombophlebitis stasis and hypercoagulability are present in all pregnancies. There are two types of thrombophlebitis/thrombus: superficial and deep vein. Superficial venous thrombus usually involves the saphenous veins and is confined to the lower leg. It is often seen in women who have varicose veins. Deep venous thrombus can involve any veins from the foot to the iliofemoral region; it predisposes the client to pulmonary embolism.

Risk Factors

- Postpartum immobility
- Cesarean birth
- Pregnancy-induced hypertension (PIH)
- Varicose veins
- Smoking
- Diabetes mellitus
- Excessive fluid loss and dehydration
- Hydramnios
- Women over 40 years old

- Multiparity
- Anemia
- Heart disease

Signs and Symptoms

Superficial venous thrombus occurs three to four days postpartum—reddened, warm, swollen over clot area. Leg is tender to touch but the clot is firmly attached to the vein.

Deep vein thrombosis occurs in larger veins; thrombus can break away forming an embolus. Symptoms of deep vein thrombosis are: pain, low-grade fever, chills, swelling and paleness of affected leg, and positive Homan's sign.

Diagnostic Tests and Labs

- Homan sign—calf pain elicited on dorsiflexion of the foot
- Ultrasound or computed tomography (CT scan) to visualize clot
- Venography
- Impedance plethysmography
- Clotting times (to regulate anticoagulant therapy)
- Prothrombin or partial prothrombin times (to regulate anticoagulant therapy)

Therapeutic Nursing Management

- Provide bed rest with leg elevated; change positions frequently.
- Client should not place knees in a sharply flexed position.
- Teach to avoid rubbing affected area.
- Teach the client to avoid prolonged sitting
- Take daily measurements of calf and thigh circumference.
- Apply support stockings.
- Apply moist heat applications.
- Preventive measures: early ambulation, adequate hydration (at least 2,500 mL daily).
- For clients on heparin, monitor for signs of hemorrhage (e.g., bruising, petechiae, blood in urine, bleeding gums, increased vaginal bleeding, tachycardia, and falling blood pressure).
- Teaching home care for clients taking anticoagulants:
  - Avoid aspirin and nonsteroidal anti-inflammatory drugs (which increase the risk of hemorrhage).
  - Do not go barefoot.
  - Brush teeth gently with soft toothbrush.
  - Postpone dental appointments.
  - Do not use a razor to shave legs and underarms.
  - Avoid use of alcohol (inhibits the metabolism of warfarin).

- Report any side effects, such as unexplained fever, sore throat, or fatigue (signs of agranulocytosis).

Pharmacologic Management

- Analgesics
- Anticoagulants (intravenous heparin, oral warfarin). Protamine sulfate is the antidote for heparin; vitamin K is the antidote for warfarin.

Complications

Embolism occurs when a deep vein thrombosis breaks loose and travels through the pulmonary circulation. Signs and symptoms of pulmonary embolism include: syncope, respiratory arrest, sharp stabbing chest pain, dyspnea, auscultation of crackles, hypotension, tachycardia, diaphoresis, pallor, cyanosis, hemoptysis, and anxiety.

Critical Thinking Exercise: Nursing Management of the Client with Thrombophlebitis

Situation: Two postpartum clients have venous thrombosis. Client A has a history of varicose veins; her left leg has two warm, tender, red areas along the medial calf of her leg. The vein in that area is enlarged and hard, and the client says it hurts when she walks. Client B has pain in her left leg when she ambulates, and she says her leg "feels stiff." Her calf is swollen and her foot is edematous. Her leg is pale and cool to the touch, and the pedal and posterior tibial pulses are diminished.

1. Which client has superficial venous thrombosis?

2. How is the care of these two clients similar?

3. Which client is at most risk for a pulmonary embolus?

4. What nursing interventions will Client B need that are not needed by Client A? Why?

5. How would Client B's treatment be different if she were pregnant? Why?

Nursing Management of the Client with Postpartum Blues

> ## Key Points
>
> - Postpartum blues (baby blues) are normal; up to 80% of women experience this.
> - Symptoms of postpartum blues peak at about five days postpartum and subside within two weeks.
> - The cause of postpartum blues is unknown; etiologies may include biochemical, psychological, and sociocultural factors.
> - Depressive symptoms can interfere with maternal role attainment.
> - Nurses should teach women how to differentiate between postpartum blues and the more severe postpartum depression.
> - **Key Terms/Concepts**: Postpartum blues, baby blues, postpartum depression, client/ family teaching

Overview

It is estimated that as many as 80% of women experience a "blue" period during the first two weeks after the birth of a baby. Although postpartum blues, or "baby blues," are usually mild and over soon, up to 15% of women experience the more severe postpartum depression, which can cause the woman to have feelings of guilt, failure, loneliness, and low self-esteem.

Etiologies

- The cause of postpartum blues is unknown, although biochemical, psychological, social, and cultural factors have all been suggested.
- Physical factors may include the lower level of circulating glucocorticoids and subclinical hypothyroidism that may exist in the early postpartum period. The fatigue of childbirth and the fatigue caused by the demands of the new baby may also be physical causes.
- Psychologically, the new mother may be overwhelmed by parental responsibilities, feel a loss at the separation of baby and self, and feel a lack of the attention and support that existed during pregnancy.

Signs and Symptoms of Postpartum Blues

- Emotional lability (e.g., crying easily and for no apparent reason)
- Depression
- A feeling of being let down
- Restlessness
- Fatigue, insomnia

- Headache
- Anxiety
- Anger
- Sadness
- Symptoms peak at around five days postpartum and subside by the tenth day.
- Symptoms are mild

Risk Factors for Postpartum Depression

- High level of anxiety during pregnancy
- Ambivalence about whether to terminate or maintain the pregnancy
- Discord in the marital relationship
- Previous experiences of postpartum depression
- Inadequate support system (e.g., extended family, friends)
- Family history of abuse, neglect, and/or alcoholism
- Low income level
- History of premenstrual syndrome (PMS)

Therapeutic Nursing Management

- At postpartum visits, screen all women for risk factors of postpartum depression.
- Assure the woman that "baby blues" are normal.
- Help her plan strategies for getting rest (e.g., nap when the baby does; go to bed early; let the housework go).
- Teach the woman to nurture herself (e.g., go for a walk or read a book while family members care for the baby).
- Suggest that the woman plan an occasional day out of the house (e.g., lunch with friends or taking the baby in a stroller to go shopping).
- Encourage the woman to tell her partner how she feels.
- Teach women how to recognize postpartum depression (PPD):
  - Severe symptoms, symptoms that are still present after two weeks, or symptoms that begin after two weeks postpartum
  - Several of the symptoms are present every day
  - Depression, sadness, and spontaneous crying
  - Withdrawal, even while complaining about lack of support from partner and others
  - Sleep disorders (e.g., inability to go back to sleep after infant feedings)
  - Extreme fatigue, to the point of interfering with functioning
  - Appetite change; weight increase or decrease
  - Feelings of worthlessness or guilt
  - Difficulty concentrating
  - Fears for the baby
  - Thoughts of suicide

- A variety of PPD scales exist, which can be used to evaluate the severity and frequency of a woman's symptoms (e.g., the Beck Postpartum Depression Checklist and the Edinburgh Postnatal Depression Scale).
- A referral for professional mental health assessment and antidepressant therapy may be indicated.

Complications

- Postpartum depression
- Delayed maternal role attainment
- Delayed maternal-infant bonding

Critical Thinking Exercise: Nursing Management of the Client with Postpartum Blues

Situation: C.C. gave birth to a healthy, full-term baby girl after a somewhat difficult pregnancy. She was not married when she became pregnant, and at 10 weeks' gestation, she considered having an abortion. Her parents urged her to continue the pregnancy and marry the baby's father, which she did. However, even at her last prenatal visit, she was still anxious about the limitations that a baby would impose on her. Shortly before the birth, her husband was imprisoned for stealing a car. C.C. is unemployed and living on public aid; her parents do not have room in their trailer for her and the baby.

Five days after the birth of her baby, a home health nurse is visiting C.C. Her hair has not been combed and her body odor suggests that she has not been bathing. The nurse sees that the house is messy and dirty. When asked how she is doing, C.C. starts crying. She says, "I'm just so tired; and there's no one to help me. I am so mad at my parents for talking me into this!"

1. What data in C.C.'s history should alert the nurse that she is at risk for postpartum depression?

2. What symptoms of postpartum blues is C.C. exhibiting at this time? Which symptoms should be explored as possible symptoms of postpartum depression?

3. What other information does the nurse need in order to determine whether C.C.'s symptoms are normal or whether she may have postpartum depression?

4. How can the nurse help C.C. at this time?

Physical Assessment Norms

> ## Key Points
>
> - The first assessment, performed at birth, includes Apgar scoring and a quick check for serious abnormalities.
> - A complete physical examination is done within 24 hours, after the temperature stabilizes.
> - A complete assessment includes general appearance, vital signs, measurements, and head-to-toe assessment.
> - Posture should be flexed.
> - Fontanels should be palpable.
> - Molding of the head may cause the head to appear misshapen, but it is normal.
> - Respirations 30-60/min; heart rate 120-160/min; 100 during sleep and 180 when crying.
> - Head should be larger than chest.
> - Umbilical cord has two arteries and one vein.
> - Reflexes: Rooting, sucking, grasp, Moro, startle, Babinski, step, and tonic neck (fencing).
> - **Key Terms/Concepts**: Lanugo, vernix caseosa, acrocyanosis, erythema toxicum, Mongolian spots, harlequin sign, apnea, fontanel, milia, strabismus, nystagmus

Overview

The newborn undergoes numerous biologic changes in making the transition to extrauterine life. Although most infants make the necessary adjustments, the first 24 hours are critical because respiratory distress and circulatory failure can occur rapidly and almost without warning.

Assessment begins at birth, with assignment of an Apgar score. A complete physical examination should be done after the baby's temperature stabilizes, within 24 hours of birth. A complete newborn physical assessment includes: general appearance, vital signs, measurements, and head-to-toe assessment. Data may be recorded on special forms or as descriptive notes.

General Appearance

- Posture—flexed with good muscle tone
- Skin—soft; smooth; good turgor; possible peeling and dryness of hands and feet; pink- to-ruddy color; lanugo may be present on face, brow, shoulders; vernix in folds; acrocyanosis; erythema toxicum, Mongolian spots, and harlequin sign are normal variations.

- Color/Perfusion–brisk capillary refill (approximately two seconds) with pink-to-ruddy color (no pallor or dusky appearance).

Vital Signs and Measures

Respiratory rate: 30-60 per minute; short periods of periodic breathing patterns, passing tachypnea. Breath sounds clear. Respirations are shallow and irregular. Breathing is abdominal and movements are symmetric.

Heart rate: 110-160 per minute; ranges from 180 when crying to 100 during sleep. Blood pressure: 70/45 during the first 36 hours in quiet, alert state (blood pressure is not routinely taken).

Temperature: 36.5-37.5° C (97.5-99.3° F). Axillary temperature is preferred. One rectal temperature may be done to assess for patency of the anus.

Weight: 5 lb. 8 oz-8 lb. 13 oz; weight loss of five to 10% normal in first few days. Should return to birth weight by first week.

Length: 45-55 cm (17.75-21.5 inches)

Head circumference: 31-38 cm (12.2-15 inches)

Chest circumference: 31-36 cm (12.2-14.2 inches)

Head-to-Toe Assessment

Head

- Vaginal birth—molding evident; cesarean birth—well-rounded, unless labor preceded surgical intervention
- Anterior and posterior fontanels palpable, flat and soft
- No bruising, abrasions or swelling
- Sagittal suture may be overlapping fingertip spread
- Cephalhematoma or caput present or absent

Face

- Symmetrical facial movement
- Milia over nose, chin
- Nares patent bilaterally
- Mouth—midline, symmetric, mucous membranes pink, Epstein pearl may be noticed
- Eyes symmetric, slate blue, dark gray or brown; sclera white to bluish white; strabismus and nystagmus possible
- Ear pinna recoils; placement in line with eyes; abnormal shape, placement or rotation should be documented

Neck

- Short
- Symmetric
- Supple

Chest

- Round, symmetric, slightly smaller than head
- Areola stippled, raised
- No crepitation; clavicles intact

Abdomen

- Protrudes, no distention
- Umbilical cord has two arteries, one vein
- Bowel sounds present
- Passing meconium/patent anus

Genitals

- Female—labia majora covers clitoris and labia minora in the term infant; vaginal opening patent; may have vaginal discharge
- Male—penis straight without chordae; testes palpable in scrotum; urethral opening at the end of penis

Extremities

- Symmetric, flexed; nail beds pink
- Three creases in palm, one continuous crease across palm is a finding associated with Down Syndrome
- No creases on plantar surface
- Spine—straight, at midline; no sacral dimple or tuft of hair
- Hips—no "clunk" noted with manipulation of hips

Reflexes present

- **Rooting**—seen when the cheek is stroked and newborn responds with a turn of the head toward the touch
- **Sucking**—well-developed at birth
- **Grasp**—pressure on the palms of the hands or soles of the feet causes flexion of fingers or toes
- **Moro**—immediate, bilateral, symmetric response to sudden jarring or abrupt change in equilibrium; diminishes by six months of age
- **Startle**—similar to Moro. Consists of abduction of arms and flexion of elbows following loud noise
- **Babinski**—when plantar lateral surface of neonate's foot is stroked the toes flare. Disappears at one year.
- **Step, dance reflex**—until six weeks, when held in an upright position, neonate makes stepping movements
- **Tonic neck**—fencing reflex; when newborn lies on the back with head turned to one side, the arm and leg on the same side are extended, and the opposite arm is flexed; disappears three to four months of age

Senses

- **Vision**— normal term infant sees clearly nine to 12 inches away from eyes, 30 degrees either way from midline

- **Hearing**—newborns turn toward sound; can discriminate parents' voices; mother preferred
- **Taste**—can taste; prefers sweet over salty
- **Smell**—highly sensitive sense of smell; newborns exhibit physiologic change when exposed to strong odors
- **Touch**—very sensitive to touch and pain

Critical Thinking Exercise: Physical Assessment Norms

1. Match the descriptions to the correct newborn reflex.

a.	When the nurse strokes the infant's palate, he begins to suck.		Babinski
b.	When the nurse strokes the infant's cheek, the infant turns her head to that side.		Grasp
c.	The infant's toes flare outward and the big toe dorsiflexes when the nurse strokes the lateral sole of its foot.		Moro
d.	When the nurse raises the infant and then allows the head and trunk to drop back 30 degrees, the infant's arms and legs extend and abduct, the fingers fan open with the thumbs and forefingers forming a "C"; the arms then return to their normally flexed state.		Rooting
e.	When the nurse claps her hands near the infant, the infant abducts the arms and flexes the elbows, similar to a Moro reflex.		Startle
f.	When the nurse touches the baby's palm near the base of the fingers, the hand closes into a tight fist.		Step
g.	When the nurse holds the infant upright with the feet touching the bed, the infant lifts one foot and then the other.		Sucking
h.	When lying on the back with head turned to one side, the infant extends the arm and leg on the same side and flexes the opposite arm.		Tonic neck

2. Which of the following newborns is not breathing normally? (There may be more than one.)

   Baby A is breathing deeply, with a regular rhythm, at a rate of 40/min.
   Baby B is sleeping. He is breathing shallowly, at a rate of 26/min, with short periods of apnea.
   Baby C is sleeping. He is breathing diaphragmatically and his sternum is retracting. The rate is 70/min.
   Baby D is crying. He is breathing abdominally, irregularly, and at a rate of 70/min.
   Baby E is breathing shallowly, with 40-second periods of apnea and cyanosis.

3. Why does the nurse need to count a newborn's apical pulse and respirations for a full minute?

Situation: A newborn (4 hours old) weighs 8 lb. and is 20 inches long. Her head is 12 inches in circumference and her chest is 14 inches in circumference. Her anterior fontanel is palpable; the posterior fontanel is not. Bowel sounds are present and she has just passed meconium. She has fine hair on her forehead and shoulders and vernix in the folds of her wrists, elbows, and ankles.

4. Why is it significant that the infant has passed meconium?

5. Which of the assessment findings may be cause for concern?

Apgar Assessment

> ## Key Points
>
> - Apgar scoring assesses the newborn's cardiorespiratory adaptation at birth.
> - The Apgar score is determined at one and five minutes after birth.
> - The total score ranges from 1 to 10.
> - The indicators scored are: heart rate, respiratory effort, muscle tone, reflex irritability, and skin color.
> - A score of 8 to 10 is good; five to seven requires stimulation and oxygen; 0 to four requires resuscitation
> - **Key Terms/Concepts**: Cardiorespiratory adaptation, one minute/five minute, five indicators.

Overview

The Apgar scoring system is a means of assessing the cardiorespiratory adaptation of the newborn immediately after birth. The Apgar score is determined at one, five minutes and ten minutes. The Apgar score is based on five indicators of health: heart rate, respiratory effort, muscle tone, reflex irritability, and skin color. Each of the five indicators is scored as 0, one, or two; the scores are added to obtain a total score that can range from 0 to 10. The five minute scores are more indicative of neonatal transition to extrauterine life than the one minute assignments.

General Appearance

- The indicators are arranged from most important (heart rate) to least important.
- Heart rate: absent = 0; below 100 = one; above 100 = two
- Respiratory rate: absent = 0; slow irregular = one; good crying = two
- Muscle tone: limp = 0; some flexion of extremities = one; active motion = two
- Reflex irritability: no response to stimuli = 0; grimace = one; cough or sneeze = two
- Color: blue/pale = 0; body pink, extremities blue = one; completely pink = two

Therapeutic Nursing Management

- Each of the five indicators is rated 0 to two.
- The total score (0 to 10) is used to determine neonatal health: 8 to 10 is good; 5 to 7 means special attention may be required (e.g., gently stimulate by rubbing the infant's back; administer oxygen); 0 to four indicates serious respiratory and cardiovascular depression requiring immediate intervention, such as incubation, oxygen, or cardiopulmonary resuscitation.

Critical Thinking Exercise: Apgar Assessment

1. A baby boy was born at 12:15 p.m. At 12:16, the nurse obtains an Apgar score of 8. When should the next Apgar assessment be performed?

2. One minute after birth an infant's heart rate is 60/min. The baby has slow respirations and a weak cry, slight flexion of extremities, grimaces when suctioned, and is pink except for the hands and feet, which are blue. What is the Apgar score?

3. What nursing intervention is required for the infant in the preceding question?

4. When assessed at five minutes after birth, the infant's heart rate is 110/min. The baby now has a strong cry, but still has minimal flexion of the extremities. The baby moves promptly when slapped gently on the sole of the foot. Color is unchanged: pink except for acrocyanosis. What is the 5-minute Apgar score?

5. What nursing intervention is now required?

Newborn Care after Delivery

Key Points

- The most critical adjustments for the newborn to make immediately after birth are:
  - Establishing respirations
  - Making cardiovascular adaptations
  - Establishing thermoregulation
- Nursing care focuses on monitoring and supporting adjustments to extrauterine adaptation.
- Safety measures include matching identification bracelets for the mother and infant, footprinting the infant, and thumbprinting the mother.
- **Key Terms/Concepts**: ABCs, aquamephyton (vitamin K), opthalmic ointment (antibiotic), hepatitis B, vaccine, identification bands

Overview

Nursing care includes physical support of the neonate immediately after delivery. The most critical adjustment for the newborn is the establishment of respirations and maintaining an adequate oxygen supply (circulation). The second most critical factor is thermoregulation. Therapeutic measures in this section refer to those provided immediately after birth, although many continue until the infant goes home.

Therapeutic Nursing Management

- Suction mouth and then the nose. Stimulate cry by drying.
- Provide warmth. Put on hat because a great deal of heat loss can occur through the scalp.
- Assess respiratory effort, heart rate, color, muscle tone, and irritability; and examine physical characteristics.
- Take baby's axillary temperature (no longer any evidence for rectal temperature nor are many institutions doing this).
- Assess the cord for three vessels.
- Perform gestational age assessment.
- Assign Apgar scores (at one minute and five minutes).
- Weigh and measure.
- Fit mother and newborn with matching identification bracelets.
- Take newborn's footprint and the mother's thumbprint.
- After temperature stabilizes, bathe infant.
- Position infant on his back to sleep.

Pharmacologic Management

- Administer vitamin K (aquamephyton) intramuscularly to prevent bleeding problems until infant can produce its own clotting factors.
- Administer antibacterial agent to eyes to prevent ophthalmia neonatorum.
  - Ilotycin ointment (erythromycin 0.5%)
  - Tetracycline ointment 1%
  - Administer Hepatitis B immunization per nursery protocol or medical order. Obtain informed consent for immunization prior to injection. Document on the immunization record.

To Administer Eye Ointment

- Clean newborn's eyelids with sterile water.
- Open eyelid and apply ophthalmic antibiotic ointment.
- Do not rinse eyelids.
- Wipe excess medications from eyelid and surrounding area.
- Note: Some infants develop a mild inflammation after prophylactic treatment of the eyes.
- Note: The medication temporarily blurs the infant's vision; parents may wish to delay treatment during the initial bonding period.
- Silver nitrate solution 1% is no longer recommended for prophylaxis or treatment of congenital eye infection because of the irritation to the conjunctiva.

Complications

- Hypothermia
- Respiratory distress
- Breach of safety (identification, abduction)

Critical Thinking Exercise: Newborn Care after Delivery

Situation: A baby girl has just been born. She is full term and weighs 7 lb, 8 oz. Her Apgar score is 8 at one minute.

1. Prioritize the following nursing activities in the immediate care of the baby.

    _____ Place the infant skin-to-skin with the mother, in a warmer, or use any other method to prevent heat loss.

    _____ Support respiratory adaptation: suction the mouth and then the nose.

    _____ Perform a complete physical examination.

    _____ Bathe the infant.

    _____ Administer Ilotycin eye ointment.

    _____ Assess the baby's respirations and heart rate.

    _____ Footprint the baby and thumbprint the mother; apply matching identification bracelets.

2. Write nursing interventions to help achieve the following goals for the infant:

    a. Respiratory adaptation:

    b. Safety, including prevention of infection:

    c. Thermoregulation:

3. The parents ask you to explain the purpose of the eye ointment and vitamin K. How would you describe the reason for their administration?

Newborn Temperature Regulation

Key Points

- Thermoregulation is the maintenance of balance between heat produced and heat lost to the environment.
- The newborn is at risk for hypothermia primarily because of excessive heat loss rather than impaired heat production.
- Minimizing heat loss in the newborn is essential.
- Hypothermia increases the basal metabolic rate, resulting in increased oxygen consumption.
- Nursing interventions focus on monitoring the temperature and preventing heat loss (e.g., by controlling the environmental temperature and placing a cap on the newborn's head).
- **Key Terms/Concepts**: Thermoregulation, thermogenesis, nonshivering, brown fat, evaporation, convection, conduction, radiation, thermal neutral zone

Overview

Thermoregulation is defined as controlling heat production,   the balance between heat loss and heat production. Normal temperature of a newborn is 36.5° C (97.7° F), with a normal range of 36.5 to 37.5° C (97.7 to 98.6° F). Although newborns can produce heat fairly well, they have a tendency to lose heat rapidly in a cold environment. This is because the newborn has a large body surface in relation to body mass, less subcutaneous fat, and a thinner epidermis than an adult. Because the blood vessels are closer to the skin, the circulating blood is influenced by changes in environmental temperature.

Thermogenesis is heat production. Because newborns cannot shiver to produce heat, the main source of heat for them is "brown fat," which produces intense lipid metabolic activity. Premature, post-term, and small-for-gestational-age infants are at risk for cold stress because they lack brown fat.

Mechanisms of heat loss include:

- Evaporation: Heat loss that occurs when a liquid is converted to a vapor (e.g., when water evaporates from the skin)
- Convection: Heat loss that occurs from the flow of heat from the body surface to cooler ambient air. This is why room temperatures should not be too cool.
- Conduction: Heat loss from the body surface to cooler surfaces with which it is in direct contact. This is why the newborn is placed on a warmed crib at first.

- Radiation: Heat lost from the body surface to a cooler solid surface that is nearby, but not in direct contact with the body. This is why the newborn's crib is not placed close to a cool window.

Risk Factors for Cold Stress

- Small for gestational age (SGA)
- Prematurity
- Post-dates
- Large for gestational age (LGA)
- Precipitous delivery
- Delayed drying
- Placement on a cold surface or cool, drafty area
- Disruption in the skin integrity (gastroschisis, omphalocele or myelomeningocele)

Signs and Symptoms—Cold Stress

- Cool extremities
- Lethargy
- Apnea
- Tachypnea
- Poor feeding
- Nasal flaring
- Grunting
- Retractions

Therapeutic Nursing Management

- Maintain neutral thermal environment for the newborn—an environment in which the newborn's metabolic rate and oxygen consumption are minimal and internal body temperature is maintained because of thermal balance. For a full-term unclothed newborn, this is a room temperature of 89.6 to 93.2° F (32 to 34° C).
- Dry the neonate with warm blankets after birth.
- Keep newborn's head dry and covered.
- Protect newborn from drafts.
- Maintain warm environment until body temperature stabilizes (e.g., radiant warmer).
- Warm oxygen before administration.
- Protect newborn from conduction heat loss (e.g., use a blanket on the scale).
- Encourage skin-to-skin contact with mother.
- Preheat all equipment used on newborn.

- Perform all procedures quickly, expose skin only as necessary, and rewrap infant immediately.

Complications

- Cold stress causes increased metabolism, leading to hypoxia, acidosis, and respiratory distress.
- Cold stress further compromises a newborn with other physiologic problems.
- If cold stress is not corrected, it may lead to newborn shock, respiratory distress, metabolic acidosis, disseminated intravascular coagulopathy (DIC), or death.

Critical Thinking Exercise: Newborn Temperature Regulation

1. Match the nursing interventions to the mechanism of heat loss they are meant to prevent.

Mechanism of Heat Loss		
	a.	Regulate room temperature to keep it in the thermal neutral zone.
Conduction	b.	Keep a hat on the newborn's head.
Convection	c.	Dry the infant well after birth.
Evaporation	d.	Warm hands and stethoscope before touching baby.
Radiation	e.	Do not place crib close to a window or fan.
	f.	Dry the baby well when bathing.
	g.	Keep the infant well wrapped.
	h.	Use a warm blanket to wrap the infant.
	i.	Place infant skin-to-skin with mother when feeding.

Situation: A baby was born one hour ago after a precipitous birth. He weighed 7 lb. 8 oz. The baby's heart rate is 120 and respirations are 38. Auxiliary temperature, taken just after birth, was 98° F. The mother is holding the loosely wrapped baby, counting fingers and toes, and so on. The baby is lying with flexed arms and legs, and is not shivering. The mother points out to the nurse that the baby's hands and feet are blue.

2. What should the nurse do? Why?

3. What risk factors for hypothermia are present in the environment?

Nursing Management of the Newborn's Nutritional Needs

Key Points

- A normal newborn requires 100-120 kcal/kg/day.
- An infant's daily fluid intake should be about 100-150 mL/kg/day.
- Human milk is the most complete food available for the newborn.
- Commercial formulas can provide adequate nutrition.
- Both human milk and commercial formulas supply adequate amounts of most vitamins.
- Cow's milk lacks vitamin C.
- Solid foods (e.g., cereal, egg yolk, meat) are introduced at age six months to supply iron.
- Regurgitation ("spitting up") is common.
- **Key Term/Concepts**: Non-nutritive sucking, caloric/fluid requirements, client teaching

Overview

Sufficient protein, fluid, minerals, and vitamins to support normal growth and development meet a newborn's nutritional needs. Normal, full-term newborns require 100-120 kcal/kg/day. Carbohydrates should provide the main energy source. Protein is used for tissue growth. Fats provide additional energy and essential fatty acids for growth and health. The most complete food available for the infant is human milk; however, commercially-prepared formulas can provide adequate nutrition. Formula-fed infants usually eat every three to four hours; breastfed infants may eat more frequently.

- Carbohydrates: Because the newborn has small glycogen stores, it is important that carbohydrates be given at frequent intervals. Lactose is the primary carbohydrate.
- Fats: About 15% of the infant's intake should come from fats. Fats provide fatty acids needed for growth and cell structures.
- Protein: Supplies the basic growth element of the body. Providing essential amino acids, protein is found in milk and the mixed infant diet. During the first six months, an infant requires 2.2 g/kg per day of protein. During the second six months, daily requirement drops to 2.0 g/kg/day.
- Water: An essential requirement for life. An infant's body weight is 70-75% water. The approximate daily infant need for water is 150 mL/kg/day. Both formula and breast milk contain enough water if the infant is feeding well.

- Minerals: Essential in overall metabolism. Calcium and iron are particularly important in general infant nutrition. Calcium is essential for rapid bone mineralization, muscle contraction, blood coagulation, nerve irritability, tooth development, and heart muscle action. Milk satisfies infant's need for calcium. Iron is an essential trace element necessary for the synthesis of hemoglobin. A six-month supply of iron is stored in the fetal liver. The infant needs solid foods to supply iron at about 6 months. Enriched cereal, egg yolk, and meat provide iron.
- Vitamins: Both human and cow's milk provide adequate amounts of most vitamins, especially A and the B-complex. Cow's milk lacks vitamin C. Commercially-prepared formulas are fortified with vitamin C. Vitamin K is given as an injection at the time of delivery. After that, it is synthesized by intestinal bacterial flora.

Therapeutic Nursing Management

- Teach basic nutritional needs. Provide education regarding the normal needs for foods by six months.
- Teach breast- or bottle-feeding techniques.
- Teach the parents that infants take about an ounce of formula at a time during the first day or two, increasing to two to three ounces per feeding in the first two weeks. By age 12 weeks, they are usually drinking five to six ounces at a feeding (every three to four hours). When the fluid intake exceeds 32-36 ounces/day, the infant may require supplemental feeding with an iron- fortified rice cereal. However, the infant will need to demonstrate effective swallowing and lack of extrusion reflex. When bottle feeding, the baby should be held close with the head upright. The bottle should be held such that there is no air in the nipple. The infant should be burped frequently to avoid regurgitation. Any unused formula should be discarded and not refrigerated for reuse.
- Teach breastfeeding mothers that feeding time varies, but generally should last at least 15 minutes initially. The feeding should be ended when the infant falls asleep or after a short period of non-nutritive sucking.
- Instruct parents to breast or bottle feed with commercial formula until the baby is 12 months old.

Complications

- Malnutrition—specific to deficit
- Failure to thrive
- Iron deficiency anemia due to not receiving supplemental iron with cow's milk

Critical Thinking Exercise: Nursing Management of the Newborn's Nutritional Needs

Situation: An average newborn infant weighs 8 lbs (3.64 kg).

1. How many calories per day does this baby need?

2. If formula contains 20 kcal/ounce, how many ounces of formula will the newborn need per day?

3. If the newborn takes exactly two ounces at each feeding, how many feedings will be needed in order to take in 18-22 ounces (or the necessary number of calories)? Over a 24-hour period, how often would the baby need to eat?

4. A new mother asks you to describe how much breast milk her baby is getting at a feeding and if it is enough for this infant. She explains that her mother who did not breastfeed is worried. How will you answer? How would your answer be different on Day 3 or at two weeks of age?

Nursing Management of the Newborn with a Circumcision

Key Points

- Circumcision is an elective procedure.
- Parents should be given adequate information to make an informed choice.
- The main immediate post-procedural complication is hemorrhage.
- Other complications include infection and stenosis.
- It is important to comfort the baby during and after the procedure.
- Post-procedure interventions include keeping petroleum jelly on the site and protecting the site from pressure.
- The yellow exudate that forms on the second day should not be removed; it is not a sign of infection.
- **Key Terms/Concepts:** Gomco, Plastibell, parent teaching, hemorrhage

Overview

Circumcision is a voluntary, elective, surgical procedure that removes the foreskin from the penis. There are different points of view regarding circumcision. Benefits include possible prevention of such diseases as urinary tract infection and cancer of the penis. Risks include potential post-procedure bleeding and infection. The family, on the basis of cultural, social, and family traditions usually makes the decision. Frequently-stated reasons are that they want to (a) have the male child look like the father or brothers, and (b) prevent the need for a more painful experience should circumcision become necessary later in life. The American Academy of Pediatrics recommends against circumcision; they also suggest that analgesia be used during the procedure to reduce pain.

Pharmacology/Analgesia

- 1% lidocaine for dorsal penile nerve block
- Acetaminophen
- Cryoanalgesia
- Topical anesthetics/creams

Therapeutic Nursing Management

- Before the procedure be sure the parents understand the procedure; answer any questions; and be sure that an informed consent is signed.
- Check for family history of bleeding disorders and mothers who took anticoagulants during pregnancy (including aspirin).

- During the procedure, comfort the baby by stroking his head, talking to him, and/or giving him a pacifier.
- Give infant to parents as soon as possible after the procedure, to allow them to comfort the infant and relieve their anxiety. Teach them to observe for signs of over stimulation (turning away his head, increased generalized body movement, skin color changes, hyperalertness, and hiccuping).
- Observe for bleeding every 15 to 30 minutes for two hours after the procedure (depending on agency policy).
- If bleeding is heavy, apply intermittent light pressure to the site with a sterile gauze pad; call the primary care provider.
- Position infant on side after the procedure, and fasten diaper loosely to prevent pressure on the site.
- Advise parents that the baby may be fussy and not feed as well for several hours after the procedure.

Parent Education

- Cleanse penis during bath and with each diaper change (squeeze water over the penis and pat it dry).
- Avoid tub baths until circumcision is healed.
- Use petroleum jelly or A & D ointment on circumcision site until it is well healed (unless Plastibell was used); this keeps the diaper from adhering to the site.
- Observe site for bleeding or discharge with foul odor.
- Recognize signs of infection and report to clinician.
- Expect circumcision will be completely healed at two weeks.
- Do not remove the small yellow exudate that may be seen on the second day.
- If a Plastibell is used, it should fall off within eight days. If not, notify the primary care provider.

Early Postprocedural Complications

- Pain
- Restlessness
- Hemorrhage
- Infection
- Difficulty voiding
- Dehiscence

Later Complications

- Meatitis
- Adhesion
- Fistula
- Stenosis
- Ulcerations

Critical Thinking Exercise: Nursing Management of the Newborn with a Circumcision

Situation: The parents of a newborn male infant have been asked if they wish to have their baby circumcised. They seem anxious and tell the nurse, "We don't really know if we should do this. We are afraid it will hurt him. Does he need to have it done?"

1. What nursing diagnosis is most appropriate?

2. How can the nurse help decrease the parents' anxiety?

3. The parents decide to have the baby circumcised. One hour after the procedure, they call the nurse to their room to show her a 1 x 2 cm spot of blood on the dressing covering the site. What should the nurse do?

4. Three hours after the circumcision, the parents again call the nurse. This time there is a 2 x 2 inch spot of blood on the dressing. What should the nurse do?

5. The baby is dismissed to home care after 24 hours. The next day, the parents telephone the primary care provider's office to report that the baby's penis has "some yellow stuff" on it. They say that it is not bleeding and that they have been keeping petroleum jelly on the site, as instructed. When asked, they say that the yellow exudate does not have any odor. They ask, "What should we do? Try to wash it off? Bring him to see the doctor? What?" What should the nurse tell them?

Case Study: Circumcision of the Newborn

Situation: Twenty-four hours after delivery, and just prior to discharge, a male infant is about to undergo an elective circumcision. He has not been fed for several hours, and is restrained on a circumcision board. The procedure will be done using a Gomco clamp. The nursery nurse will provide care for the infant after the circumcision and prior to discharge.

Instructions: Identify the priority nursing interventions that should be included in the infant's post-circumcision care.

With a partner, list the discharge instructions that should be given to the mother when providing circumcision care at home and give the rationale for the action.

INSTRUCTIONS	RATIONALE

Discuss the positives and negatives of circumcision and your feelings about parents who decline circumcision.

PROS:

CONS:

Nursing Management of the Newborn who is Preterm

Key Points

- A preterm infant is one who is born before completion of 37 weeks' gestation.
- Prematurity is considered a high-risk condition.
- A preterm infant may be small (SGA), normal, or large (LGA) for gestational age.
- Severity and likelihood of problems are related to length of gestation.
- Responses (e.g., reflexes, muscle tone, arousal states) are usually weaker than those of a full-term infant.
- Goals are to meet the infant's growth and development needs and to anticipate and manage associated complications, such as respiratory distress syndrome and sepsis.
- **Key Terms/Concepts**: Self-regulation, surfactant, thermoregulation, metabolic rate, sepsis, passive immunity, basal metabolism, scarf sign, vernix caseosa, lanugo, fontanelle, cranial sutures, gavage, incubator

Overview

Approximately 8% of pregnancies are preterm (15% in low socioeconomic populations). A preterm infant is one born before the completion of 37 weeks' gestation. Problems of the preterm infant are caused by immaturity of all body systems; the fewer weeks of gestation completed, the less mature the systems, and the greater the likelihood of problems. The goals of therapy are to meet the infant's growth and development needs (e.g., nutrition) and to recognize and manage the complications (e.g., respiratory distress syndrome and sepsis) associated with prematurity.

Alterations in Physiology

- **Respiratory**: Decreased amounts of surfactant produced in the lungs, with resulting lack of pulmonary compliance and alveolar collapse leading to respiratory distress.
- **Thermoregulation**: Two factors that limit the infant's ability to produce heat are the lack of brown fat available for metabolism, and the lack of glycogen available in the liver. Factors contributing to heat loss include: (1) high ratio of body surface to body weight, (2) lack of subcutaneous fat for insulation, (3) thinner, more permeable skin, (4) open rather than flexed posture, and (5) decreased ability to constrict the superficial blood vessels.
- **Nutritional Factors**
  - Poorly developed gag reflex and incompetent esophageal cardiac sphincter
  - Small stomach capacity

- Poor ability to convert essential amino acids
- Kidney immaturity causes inability to handle formula protein.
- Decreased bile salts and pancreatic lipase cause difficulty in absorbing saturated fats.
- Deficiency of calcium and phosphorus, which are deposited primarily in the last trimester
- Inability to digest lactose
- Poor suck-swallow reflexes
- Increased basal metabolism and oxygen requirements caused by fatigue (e.g., from sucking)
- Diminished blood flow and perfusion of intestinal tract due to hypoxia and hypoxemia at birth

- **Renal**
  - Lower glomerular filtration rate (GFR)
  - Limited ability to concentrate urine or to excrete excess amounts of fluid
  - Reduced buffering capacity, predisposing to metabolic acidosis
  - Increased tendency to excrete glucose
  - Decreased ability to excrete drugs

- **Immunologic system**: The premature infant has an underdeveloped cellular immune system. Passive immunity is acquired from the mother in the last trimester; therefore, the premature infant has few antibodies at birth.

- **Neurological**: The most rapid brain growth and development occurs during the third trimester. Myelinization of the nerves begins in the second trimester and continues into adulthood. The risk of intraventricular hemorrhage (IVH) and intracranial hemorrhage (ICH) is greater in the preterm infant. This complication can lead to a compromised neurological development. The preterm baby's periods of reactivity may be delayed or absent. Preterm infants are more disorganized in their sleep-wake cycles, and are less able to attend to the human face and objects in the environment. All neurologic responses (e.g., sucking, muscle tone, arousal states) are less organized than those of a full-term infant.

Risk Factors (for Preterm Birth)

The causes of preterm labor are not completely understood. Risk factors include, but are not limited to, the following:

- Multiple gestation
- Maternal age younger than 18 or older than 35 years
- Low socioeconomic status
- Smoking more than 10 cigarettes per day
- DES exposure
- Substance abuse
- Uterine anomaly
- Polyhydramnios
- Febrile illness, pyelonephritis

- Poor maternal weight gain
- More than two first trimester abortions, or a second trimester abortion
- Previous preterm labor
- Sexually transmitted infections (e.g., trichomoniasis and chlamydia)
- Anemia
- Abdominal trauma
- History of having a cone biopsy

Signs and Symptoms of Prematurity

Special assessment tools (Ballard or Dubowitz assessments) are available for determining gestational age in preterm newborns. Physical characteristics and neuromuscular maturity vary greatly depending on the gestational age. However, in general, the following are seen:

- Pink, ruddy, acrocyanotic (report cyanosis, jaundice, or pallor)
- Decreased subcutaneous fat
- Translucent, reddened skin, with blood vessels readily visible
- Plentiful, widely-distributed lanugo
- Nails soft and short
- Ears have minimal cartilage and are pliable and folded over
- Resting position is flaccid and frog-like in appearance
- Cry is weak
- Head appears large in relation to body
- Head bones are pliable; fontanelle is smooth and flat; suture lines are prominent.
- Genitals are small; testes may be undescended. The female clitoris is prominent at lower gestational age
- Poor suck, swallow, and gag reflexes
- Jerky, generalized movements (report seizure activity, which is abnormal)
- Positive scarf sign
- Thick covering of vernix caseosa

Diagnostic Tests and Lab

These vary, depending on the gestational age and the complications that develop. The following are some examples:

- Abdominal x-ray: A/P and left lateral decubitus views
- Intake and output
- Urine pH and specific gravity
- Stools for guaiac
- Blood cultures
- Pulse oximeter
- Blood gases
- Blood sugar monitoring

Therapeutic Nursing Management

- If the infant can't be put to breast due to medical condition or gestational immaturity, advise/help the mother to pump her breasts and give the milk via gavage. Extra breast milk may be stored frozen for two to three months.
- Have a flexible feeding schedule so the baby can nurse during alert times.
- Calculate fluid requirements based on weight and urinary output; minimize fluid loss as needed through use of heat shields and humidity.
- Maintain respiratory function. In supine position, elevate head slightly but do not hyperextend neck; prone position facilitates lung expansion for effective ventilation. Maintain neutral airway position to prevent obstruction in breathing. Newborn head control and neck muscle strength is low and can contribute to potential poor airway alignment.
- Monitor for respiratory distress (e.g., cyanosis, tachypnea, retractions, grunting, nasal flaring, increased work of breathing, symmetry and depth of chest rise, apnea, rales/rhonchi).
- Ensure that gag and suck reflexes are intact before initiating oral feedings.
- Maintain neutral thermal environment to prevent hypothermia (e.g., warm and humidify oxygen, keep cap on baby's head, warm formula before feeding, use incubator or humidified radiant warmers).
- Maintain fluid and electrolyte status (e.g., calculate fluid needs based on body weight; monitor hourly intake and output; monitor urine specific gravity and pH; administer intravenous fluids). Hydration is considered adequate when the urine output is 1-3 mL/kg/hour.
  - Signs of dehydration: Sunken fontanelle, weight loss, poor skin turgor, dry oral mucous membranes, urine output less than 1-3 mL/kg/hour, urine specific gravity >1.013.
  - Signs of overhydration: Edema, excessive weight gain, and urine output small in comparison to fluid intake.
- Provide adequate nutrition.
  - Prevent fatigue during feeding (e.g., gavage instead of nipple feedings initially).
  - Feedings (nipple and gavage) are initially supplemented with intravenous therapy, depending on gestational maturity, respiratory status, and overall stability.
  - Observe for feeding intolerance (e.g., increasing gastric residuals, abdominal distention, occult blood in stools, lactose in stools, vomiting, diarrhea, visible loops of bowel).
  - Before each feeding, measure abdominal girth and auscultate for bowel sounds, and check for residual formula in the stomach.
- Prevent infection by using strict hand washing, separate equipment for each infant, limiting visitors, and maintaining strict aseptic techniques for procedures (e.g., IVs).
- Change baby's position and use sheepskin or a waterbed to prevent pressure area breakdowns on skin. A transparent, non-occlusive dressing may be beneficial to actual or potential pressure sites or areas of skin breakdown.

- Promote parent-infant attachment (e.g., give parents photographs of the baby to take home; involve parents in planning care; provide opportunities for parents to touch, hold, and talk to the baby). Sibling involvement is encouraged if children are healthy and free of infectious exposures prior to interaction with the preterm infant.

- Promote developmentally supportive care (balance the infant's need for stimuli with the infant's self-regulatory capacity). For example:

  - When handling the baby, use the hands to hold the baby's arms and legs flexed and close to the midline of the body.

  - Provide objects (e.g., a finger) for the infant to grasp during caregiving.

  - Provide non-nutritive sucking.

  - Provide kinesthetic stimuli by use of sheepskin and approved waterbeds.

  - Swaddle infant to keep extremities in flexed position, but be sure the hands can reach the face.

  - Use gentle touch; avoid sudden postural changes. Avoid stroking the infant's back, as this can overstimulate him/her.

Complications

- Respiratory distress syndrome (RDS)
- Pulmonary air leaks
- Patent ductus arteriosus (PDA)
- Apnea of prematurity (AOP)
- Intraventricular hemorrhage (IVH)
- Intracranial hemorrhage (ICH)
- Sepsis
- Necrotizing enterocolitis (NEC)
- Gastroesophageal reflux (GER)
- Cholestatic jaundice, metabolic bone disease, glucose intolerance
- Long-term complications include: retinopathy, bronchopulmonary dysplasia, pulmonary interstitial emphysema, and posthemorrhagic hydrocephalus.

Critical Thinking Exercise: Nursing Management of the Newborn who is Preterm

Situation: You are called to the birthing room to assist with the assessment of a 32-week gestation newborn and to provide care to the mother postpartum. The infants birth weight is 1,100 grams. The infant's Apgar scores are 3 at one minute and 7 at five minutes. The infant is having nasal flaring, grunting, substernal and intercostal retractions. He is flaccid, lying in a frog-like position. The baby is covered with a thick, cheesy substance and lanugo is widely distributed over his body.

1. Describe the unique characteristics of a preterm infant that you may see at this birth (list five).

2. Which of the assessment findings indicate that a complication may be developing?

3. Based on the data provided, write a nursing diagnosis for this baby.

4. Why is this baby at risk for Ineffective Thermoregulation?

5. How will maintaining a neutral thermal environment facilitate the baby's growth?

6. What treatment for Impaired Gas Exchange can contribute to development of hypothermia in this baby? What can the nurse do to prevent it?

Nursing Management of the Newborn who is Post-term

Key Points

- A post-term infant is one born after 42 weeks of gestation.
- Postmaturity is considered a high-risk condition.
- A postmature infant may be either small for gestational age (SGA) or large for gestational age (LGA), depending on how well the placenta functions during the last weeks of the pregnancy.
- Infants over 4000 g (8 lbs, 13 oz) are at risk for birth injuries or cesarean birth.
- If placental function deteriorates, the infant may be SGA, hypoxic, and malnourished.
- Nursing interventions focus on preventing complications and monitoring for changes in status.
- Common complications are hypoglycemia and hypothermia
- **Key Terms/Concepts**: LGA, SGS, hypoglycemia, hypothermic, hyperbilirubinemia

Overview

Approximately six to 12% of pregnancies are considered post-term. A post-term infant is one born at 42 weeks gestation or later. If postmaturity resulted in placental insufficiency, the infant will have a wasted appearance due to loss of subcutaneous fat and muscle mass. However, some postmature infants continue to grow in utero and are large at birth. The perinatal mortality rate is two to three times higher for postmature infants because the increased oxygen demands of the postmature fetus may not be met during labor and birth. Most deaths of postmature infants occur before or during labor. Only 1/6 occurs during the postpartum period.

Risk Factors

- Previous history of post-term delivery
- Primigravida
- Maternal age less than 25 years
- Preeclampsia
- Recent maternal weight loss
- Inaccurate gestational dating

Signs and Symptoms

- Meconium-stained amniotic fluid
- Abnormal fetal heart rate

- Prolonged labor
- Reduced subcutaneous tissue
- Pale, loose skin
- Wrinkled, macerated skin which becomes cracked and peels
- Increased alertness
- Long, curved nails
- Absence of vernix
- Mature genitals
- Hypoglycemia
- Large or small for gestational age

Diagnostic Tests and Lab

- Before birth: **Non-stress test (NST)** to determine fetal well-being
- Before birth: **Contraction stress test (CST)** to determine fetal/placental stress tolerance
- Infant: **Heel stick glucose screening** (Dextrostick or BG Chemstrip); CBC if polycythemia is suspected

Therapeutic Nursing Management

- Provide the newborn with frequent, early feedings for low blood sugar. In extreme cases, intravenous glucose may be given.
- Avoid cold stress in post-term newborns as it increases glucose demand.
- Monitor labor closely.
- Observe for signs of respiratory distress related to meconium aspiration.

Complications

- Hypoglycemia (related to poor stores of glycogen at birth)
- Hypothermia (related to little subcutaneous fat)
- Hyperbilirubinemia (related to polycythemia, secondary to inadequate oxygen in utero)
- Birth asphyxia (related to perinatal complications)
- Meconium aspiration and subsequent respiratory distress
- Birth injuries (fractured clavicle, intracranial hemorrhage, metabolic acidosis)

Critical Thinking Exercise: Nursing Management of the Newborn who is Post-term

Situation: Baby B., one hour old, was born at 42 weeks gestation as documented by ultrasound and LMP. He has loose skin with little subcutaneous fat. He has no lanugo and no vernix caseosa, but does have a great deal of hair on his head, as well as long fingernails. His skin is dry, cracked, and peeling. His skin, umbilical cord, and nails are meconium stained. The baby weighed 7 lbs at birth. His Apgar scores were 6 and 7 at one minute and five minutes, respectively.

1. Based on these data, what can you infer about placental functioning during the last weeks of pregnancy?

2. What ongoing assessments are especially important for this infant, and why?

3. What can the nurse do to help prevent hypoglycemia? Provide rationale for your answers.

Nursing Management of the Newborn who is Large for Gestational Age (LGA)

Key Points

- Large for gestational age means that the infant's weight is in the 90th percentile (or higher) for neonates of the same gestational age.

- Large for gestational age (LGA) neonates may be pre-, post-, or full-term. LGA does not necessarily mean postmature.

- Maternal diabetes is the best-known cause of LGA; however, only a small percentage of LGA newborns have diabetic mothers. The cause of LGA, in most cases, is unclear.

- The LGA infant is at risk for birth injuries, hypoglycemia, and polycythemia.

- Nursing interventions focus on assessing for birth trauma and screening for hypoglycemia and polycythemia.

- **Key Terms/Concepts**: Hypoglycemia, polycythemia, gestational age, macrosomia

Overview

The large for gestational age (LGA) neonate is one whose birth weight is higher than that of 90% of other neonates of the same gestational age. LGA babies may weigh over 4,000 grams (8 lbs., 13 oz.). They are usually full-term, although they may be preterm or post-term. A preterm baby who is also LGA may be mistaken for a full-term infant, but has the same problems as other, smaller, preterm infants. LGA infants are at increased perinatal risk because of being more likely to go through a longer labor, have a birth injury, or need a forceps, vacuum-assisted, or cesarean birth. LGA infants have more congenital heart defects and a higher mortality rate than babies who are appropriate for gestational age.

Risk Factors

- Diabetic mother
- Postmaturity
- Multiparity
- Large parents
- Erythroblastosis fetalis (hemolytic disease of the fetus and newborn caused by Rh incompatibility)
- Maternal obesity
- Previous delivery of a macrosomic newborn

Signs and Symptoms

- In pregnancy, a uterine fundal measurement >42 cm in the absence of hydramnios, and only average or smaller interior pelvic diameters
- In pregnancy, a biparietal diameter >10 cm verified by ultrasound or x-ray
- Birth weight in 90th percentile for gestational age
- Other symptoms depend on whether newborn is pre-, post-, or full-term.
- No vernix on skin/no lanugo (if post-term)
- Well-defined ear pinna, erect from head (if post-term)
- Skin thick, pale, desquamating (if post-term)
- Nails extend beyond fingertips (if post-term)
- Breast Buds >1 cm
- Genitals fully developed (if post-term)
- Hypertonic (in the presence of birth injuries)
- Mature physical findings

Therapeutic Nursing Management

- Perform a gestational age assessment for the newborn.
- Assess for signs of hypoglycemia (jitteriness, poor feeding, seizures, tachypnea, cyanosis, hypotonia).
- Provide early feedings of D5W if hypoglycemic.
- Monitor frequent blood sugars if symptomatic or at risk for hypoglycemia.
- Support mothers of infants with bruising of face or head, as they may be afraid to interact with the baby for fear of causing pain or further injury.

Complications

- Birth injuries (particularly to the clavicle), such as fractures, nerve damage (especially to the brachial plexus or facial nerve), cephalhematoma, or bruising
- Hypoglycemia—most often seen in infant of diabetic mother but all LGA infants should be screened for hypoglycemia
- Polycythemia—most often seen in infant of diabetic mother
- Respiratory distress—most often seen in infant of diabetic mother

Critical Thinking Exercise: Nursing Management of the Newborn who is Large for Gestational Age (LGA)

Situation: An obese, multiparous woman at 40 weeks of gestation has just given birth to a baby. After prolonged pushing in second stage, a forceps-assisted birth was necessary. The baby weighs 9 lbs 8 oz. (4,318 grams). The baby has marked caput succedaneum and marked bruising about the face, head, and shoulders.

1. How would you characterize this baby: preterm, term, post-term, LGA, SGA, or AGA (appropriate for gestational age)?

2. What risk factors for LGA do you find in this situation?

3. In order to plan individualized care for this baby, what information should be obtained from the mother's history?

4. From the history, the nurse determines that the mother is not diabetic, both the mother and infant have Rh-positive blood, and that there are many large people in both families. For this infant, what assessments should the nurse make?

5. Write a psychosocial nursing diagnosis for the parents of this infant.

Risk for_____

6. How is the care of this baby similar to the care of another infant of the same weight, but who is born at 42 weeks of gestation? How is it different?

Nursing Management of the Newborn who is Small for Gestational Age (SGA)

Key Points

- SGA describes an infant whose birth weight is at or below the 10th percentile or whose ponderal index is low (weight-to-length ratio).

- SGA results from failure to grow at the rate expected for the time in utero.

- SGA is a high-risk condition.

- SGA does not mean "premature." A baby who is SGA can be premature, full-term, or postmature.

- SGA infants who are born at term have mature organ systems and, therefore, a better survival rate than do premature infants (who are also small).

- SGA can be caused by anything that restricts uteroplacental blood flow: for example, maternal smoking, maternal diabetes or hypertension, intrauterine infections, and placental malformation.

- Because causes of SGA are so varied, the nurse must adapt care to meet whatever specific problems the infant demonstrates.

- Complications include: Hypoglycemia, meconium aspiration, polycythemia, and hypothermia

- **Key Terms/Concepts:** Asymetric growth restriction, hypoglycemia, symmetric growth restriction, hypothermia, hyperbilirubinemia

Overview

Small for gestational age (SGA) describes a neonate who weighs less than 90% or whose weight/size is at or below the 10th percentile for gestational age. That is, 90% of other neonates of the same age weigh more than this infant. SGA is a result of intrauterine growth restriction (IUGR). Small-for-gestational-age infants account for 1.5-2% of all births. Mortality for SGA infants is 3.4%; death rate from asphyxia is 8-10 times that for normal-weight (AGA) infants.

SGA babies are more mature than their weight would suggest. In spite of the growth retardation, a term SGA newborn is physiologically more mature than a preterm AGA infant. The term SGA newborn, although small, is less likely to have the complications of prematurity (e.g., respiratory distress syndrome and hyperbilirubinemia) and, therefore, more likely to survive than a preterm newborn.

Risk Factors

- **Maternal factors**: Primiparity, grand multiparity, multiple pregnancy, age extremes

- **Maternal disease**: Smoking, substance abuse, heart disease, sickle cell anemia, pregnancy-induced hypertension (PIH), diabetes mellitus, anemia, nephritis, severe malnutrition
- **Socioeconomic and environmental factors**: Low socioeconomic status, inadequate education, lack of prenatal care, exposure to toxins, exposure to x-rays
- **Placental factors**: Small placenta, infected areas, placenta previa, abnormal cord insertion, or thrombosis
- **Fetal factors**: Congenital infections (TORCH), congenital malformations

Signs and Symptoms

Symptoms vary according to whether the IUGR began early or late in pregnancy. IUGR affects the weight first; if it continues, the length and head size will also be affected.

Symmetric growth restriction involves the entire body; the body is proportionate and looks normally developed for size, although small. This is caused by long-term maternal conditions that are present in early pregnancy (e.g., chronic hypertension, anemia, substance abuse). The child will probably remain small throughout life and is more likely to have central nervous system complications.

Asymmetric growth restriction begins during the second half of pregnancy (e.g., from PIH). Such infants will usually "catch up" in growth if they are adequately nourished after birth.

- Signs and symptoms include:
  - Emaciated "little old man" appearance
  - Skin loose, scaling, dry and cracked
  - May be evidence of meconium staining
  - Head appears large because of the decreased size of the chest and abdomen (head- sparing effect)
  - Thin, shriveled cord
  - Decreased muscle mass
  - Sparse hair, skull sutures wide and large
  - Irritable, excessive crying
  - Hyper-alert, active, hungry

Diagnostic Tests and Lab

- **Blood Glucose Monitoring**: To screen blood sugar
- **Hematocrit**: To determine polycythemia (65% or greater)

Therapeutic Nursing Management

- Provide frequent early feedings for hypoglycemia.
- Perform gestational age assessment.
- Prevent hypothermia; use radiant warmers, incubator, drying, and wrapping.
- Monitor ambient room temperature.
- Assist in procedures to relieve polycythemia (exchange transfusion).

Complications

- Hypoglycemia– the most common metabolic complication of IUGR can produce central nervous system abnormalities, later learning disabilities, and mental retardation.
- Hypothermia from decreased muscle mass and decreased subcutaneous fat
- Perinatal asphyxia/acute and chronic hypoxia
- Respiratory distress related to aspiration of meconium
- Polycythemia– in response to inutero chronic hypoxia
- Infections– continuation of intrauterine infections
- Continued slow growth
- Increased congenital abnormalities
- Potential sleep pattern disturbances and continued difficulties for parents

Critical Thinking Exercise: Nursing Management of the Newborn who is Small for Gestational Age (SGA)

Situation: Baby G is born at 36 weeks of gestation. He is small for gestational age due to his mother's having pregnancy-induced hypertension during pregnancy. He appears long and thin, has sparse hair, a thin cord, dry skin, and a wide-eyed look - characteristics of "asymmetric" growth restriction that begins in the second half of pregnancy.

1. The following nursing diagnoses and collaborative problems are identified for Baby G. Supply their etiologies.

   • Impaired Gas Exchange related to: _____.

   • Potential Complication of SGA—Hypoglycemia related to:_____.

   • Hypothermia related to: _____.

   • Altered Nutrition: Less than Body Requirements related to:_____.

   • Risk for Altered Tissue Perfusion (or Potential Complication—Polycythemia) related to:

   _____.

   • Risk for Altered Parenting related to: _____.

2. Write goals/outcomes for each of the nursing diagnoses in #1.

3. Baby G's parents express concern that he is so "skinny." They are afraid he will always be small for his age. How should the nurse respond?

Nursing Management of the Newborn with Hypoglycemia

Key Points

- Hypoglycemia occurs when serum glucose is <40 mg/dL.
- If a value of less than 45 mg/dL is obtained on heel stick screening, a laboratory test should be ordered.
- If the screening test is less than 45 mg/dL, (a) feed the infant formula or breast milk and (b) retest until glucose readings are stable, and (c) notify pediatrician.
- Routine assessment of all newborns should include observing for symptoms of hypoglycemia.
- Early signs are jitteriness, poor muscle tone, and sweating.
- Nursing interventions focus on monitoring for signs and complications of hypoglycemia, notifying the primary care provider, implementing medical orders (e.g., intravenous glucose), and minimizing stress (e.g., keeping the infant warm).
- Untreated hypoglycemia may result in central nervous system damage or death.
- **Key Terms/Concepts:** Prematurity, IUGR, SGA, LGA, glucose levels/testing

Overview

During the birth process, the neonate expends large amounts of energy and consumes a great deal of glucose. In addition, the physiologic changes that occur at birth demand energy. After birth, though, the baby cannot rely on maternal glucose, so it is vulnerable to hypoglycemia in the first few days of life. In the absence of high-risk conditions, blood sugar gradually returns to normal after delivery, and stabilizes in four to six hours. Hypoglycemia occurs when serum blood glucose levels are abnormally low, a laboratory value of less than 40 mg/dL (45 mg/dL on reagent strip used with a heel stick). Almost any stress for example, asphyxia, infection, or hypothermia can create hypoglycemia in the newborn.

Risk Factors

- Maternal diabetes—High glucose loads are present in the infant in utero. When high blood sugar via the placenta stops abruptly at birth, the newborn experiences rapid hypoglycemia.
- Maternal preeclampsia—contributes to IUGR.
- Maternal intake of ritodrine or terbutaline
- Intrauterine growth retardation (IUGR)—uses up glycogen and fat stores because of intrauterine malnutrition.
- Prematurity—fetus is not in utero long enough to store glycogen and fat.

- Postmaturity
- Large for gestational age
- Asphyxia
- Cold stress

Signs and Symptoms

- Jitteriness or lethargy
- Poor feeding
- Vomiting
- Seizures, tremors, jerkiness
- High-pitched cry
- Apnea, irregular respirations, respiratory distress, cyanosis
- Hypotonia, poor suck
- May be asymptomatic

Diagnostic Tests

- Blood glucose (heel stick for blood)—Check within the first hour of age to screen for hypoglycemia. Normal level is 70-80 mg/dL. If glucose level is below 45 mg/dL, laboratory should determine the blood glucose level. Blood Sugar should be repeated at a.c. and p.c., as necessary.

Therapeutic Nursing Management

- Early breastfeeding or formula feeding is a major preventive measure.
- Provide early feeding of five to 10% glucose water for mild-to-moderate hypoglycemia.
- If neonate feeds poorly, begin on orogastric feedings.
- Per orders, start IV and administer dextrose intravenously for blood sugar below 25 Mg/100 mL and for infants who cannot tolerate enteric feedings.
- Minimize stresses that can add to hypoglycemia (e.g., cold stress increases glucose metabolism, so maintain a neutral thermal environment).
- Encourage non-nutritive sucking during gavage feedings.
- Encourage non-nutritive sucking to lower activity levels, reduce crying, and lower the baby's metabolic rate.
- Maintain intake and output to evaluate for osmotic diuresis and glycosuria.

Complications

- Hypothermia and respiratory distress
- Brain damage with severe hypoglycemia
- Seizures
- Death

Critical Thinking Exercise: Nursing Management of the Newborn with Hypoglycemia

Situation: Baby girl J.P. was born less than one hour ago. Her gestational age is 38 weeks and she is 10 lb 5 oz. J.P.'s mother was diagnosed with gestational diabetes at 26 weeks' gestation. The baby's first blood glucose reading is slightly under 40 mg/dL. J.P.'s heart rate is 120, her respirations are 80, and she is not flexing her arms and legs as newborns usually do. The mother intends to breastfeed J.P., but she has not yet attempted to do so.

1. What risk factor(s) for hypoglycemia are present in this situation?

2. Is the baby hypoglycemic?

3. What symptoms of hypoglycemia are present in this baby?

4. What measures are needed to treat the baby's hypoglycemia? Why?

5. Write three nursing diagnoses that should take priority at this time.

6. The mother attempts to breastfeed baby J.P., but the baby will not latch on and suck, even though the nurse has been present to assist the mother. What should the nurse do next?

7. In addition to measures to directly increase the blood glucose, how is care for baby J.P. similar to the care given to an infant who is small for gestational age?

Nursing Management of the Newborn with Hyperbilirubinemia

Key Points

- The best treatment is prevention. Prenatal identification of the fetus at risk for Rh or ABO incompatibility allows for in utero treatment and prevention of hemolytic disease of the newborn.

- The role of the perinatal nurse is to identify jaundice as soon as it is apparent and to differentiate between pathologic and physiologic jaundice.

- Suspect pathologic jaundice when jaundice occurs during the first 24-36 hours or after four days in a full-term newborn or prior to 48 hours in a preterm infant.

- Treatment includes phototherapy, infusion of albumin, and exchange transfusion.

- **Key Terms/Concepts**: Hyperbilirubinemia, pathologic jaundice, physiologic jaundice, kernicterus, hemolytic disease of the newborn, Rh incompatibility, phototherapy, exchange transfusion

Overview

Jaundice, a yellowish discoloration of the tissues, develops from the deposit of the yellow pigment, bilirubin, in fatty tissues. The newborn's serum bilirubin level normally does not exceed 3-5 mg/dL. Hyperbilirubinemia is an abnormally-high level of bilirubin in the blood. It is called pathologic jaundice when it occurs before 24 hours of life in a term infant and before 48 hours in a preterm infant (and the bilirubin levels are over 12 Mg/100mL in the term formula-fed newborn, 14 mg/dL in the breast-fed newborn, and 15 mg/dL in the preterm newborn). Pathologic jaundice is caused by conditions that cause excessive destruction of red blood cells (erythrocytes). Hyperbilirubinemia occurring as the result of normal newborn metabolism during the first week of life is called physiologic jaundice. It is never present during the first 24 hours of life, and it is considered normal in newborns. Jaundice is more common in breast-fed infants, usually because of insufficient intake. Breast milk jaundice is relatively rare. Jaundice in the nursing baby is most likely breastfeeding jaundice and is related to mild dehydration.

Fetal–Neonatal Blood Incompatibilities

Pathologic jaundice most often occurs because the mother and baby have different blood groups; the most frequent are ABO and Rh factor incompatibilities. If a person (e.g., a pregnant woman) is exposed to an incompatible blood type, then she will form antibodies against the antigens in that blood (e.g., the blood of the fetus). Exposure occurs if an antigen from the fetal blood crosses the placenta and enters the maternal bloodstream. The maternal antibodies that are formed then cross the placenta, and cause hemolysis of the fetal red blood cells.

- **ABO Incompatibility** occurs if the fetal blood type is A, B, or AB and the maternal blood type is O. Any person with type O blood naturally makes anti-A and anti-B antibodies. During pregnancy, the antibodies are transferred across the placenta to the fetus. Because anti-A and anti-B antibodies are already present in a type O mother, this incompatibility can affect even a firstborn infant. ABO incompatibility is more common than Rh incompatibility, but usually causes less severe problems.

- **Rh Incompatibility** occurs when the fetus of an Rh-negative mother inherits the dominant Rh-positive blood type from a father who is Rh-positive. A fetus begins to form red blood cells early in the pregnancy, and in 30-40% of pregnancies, these cells pass through the placenta into the mother's bloodstream. When the fetus is Rh+ and the mother is Rh-, the mother forms antibodies against the Rh antigens on the fetal blood cells. This is called **maternal sensitization**. During the first pregnancy with an Rh+ fetus, the woman may become sensitized, but not produce enough antibodies to cause lysis of fetal blood cells. Problems occur in subsequent pregnancies with an Rh+ fetus. Severe incompatibility results in fetal hemolytic anemia, which can result in **hydrops fetalis** (which includes marked anemia, cardiac decompensation, generalized edema, and hypoxia) and fetal death. The Rh-fetus of an Rh-mother is not in danger because the fetus does not have any of the antigens that stimulate the mother to produce antibodies.

Risk Factors

- Rh/ABO incompatibility (this is the most common cause of pathologic jaundice)
- Prematurity lowers levels of liver enzymes; poor bowel motility
- Excessive bruising
- Cephalohematoma
- Neonatal hepatitis
- Sepsis
- Hypoglycemia
- Polycythemia
- Hypoxia, respiratory distress
- Cold stress
- Dehydration
- Long-term total parenteral nutrition (TPN) infusion

Signs and Symptoms

- Yellow discoloration of the skin, sclera, and mucous membranes (jaundice)
- Poor feeding

Diagnostic Tests and Lab

- Bilirubin level: direct and total serum bilirubin
- Blood typing (for Rh and ABO incompatibility)
- Coombs' test

- Hemoglobin
- Reticulocyte percentage

Therapeutic Nursing Management

- Place under phototherapy lights and/or illumination blanket with eyes and genitals covered.
- For an infant under phototherapy, reposition every two hours to permit the light to reach all skin surfaces and to prevent pressure areas.
- Side effects of phototherapy include skin rash, loose stools and increased urine output. Observe for dehydration (e.g., intake and output, urine specific gravity) and perianal excoriation. Check diaper hourly.
- To check for output, weigh diapers. Weight in grams equals mL of urine.
- Provide frequent feedings (every two to three hours). If possible, do not offer water because the infant may take less milk.
- Monitor temperature and prevent hyperthermia or hypothermia.
- Assist with exchange transfusion or partial exchange, in which the infant's total blood volume is exchanged with donor blood.
- Do not apply lotion or ointment to the infant's skin as this may alter the natural protective barrier and make the infant prone to infections.

Complications

- Kernicterus: Neurologic damage resulting from deposits of unconjugated bilirubin in brain cells. Kernicterus occurs at serum bilirubin levels above 25 mg/dL in healthy term infants, at lower levels in preterm and low birth weight infants.
- Neonatal death

Critical Thinking Exercise: Nursing Management of the Newborn with Hyperbilirubinemia

Situation: E.M. is a 1-day-old, full-term newborn. She weighs 7 lbs 1 oz. (3.2 kg). She is receiving phototherapy because of jaundice secondary to ABO incompatibility. E.M. is breastfeeding, but has been sleepy and is feeding poorly. She has had several loose green stools. Her skin and mucous membranes are slightly dry, skin turgor is good, and the anterior fontanel is flat. Her urine is slightly dark.

1. Why does E.M. have loose green stools?

2. Place a "P" beside the nursing interventions that are being done because of E.M.'s **phototherapy**. Place an "H" beside the interventions that are being done to treat the **hyperbilirubinemia**. (NOTE: Some interventions may serve **both** purposes; mark them "PH.") Provide rationale for your answers.

   ____ Feed infant every 2-3 hours.

   ____ Weigh all diapers.

   ____ Check urine specific gravity.

   ____ Maintain a neutral thermal environment and prevent cold stress.

   ____ Dress infant in warm clothes and blankets when removing her from phototherapy.

   ____ Observe for lethargy, high-pitched cry, absent Moro reflex, and seizures.

   ____ Turn infant frequently.

3. What, if any, symptoms of Fluid Volume Deficit does E.M. have?

4. How could the nurse monitor E.M. for Fluid Volume Deficit?

5. During the past two hours, E.M's. has had one wet diaper with a net weight of 4 grams. (a) How many ounces of urine per hour does this represent? (b) Is this adequate output for E.M.?

   a.

   b.

6. In light of the information about E.M. output, what should the nurse do?

7. What nursing diagnoses should the nurse use for E.M.? For her parents?

8. Provide etiologies for the following nursing diagnoses for E.M.

   Fluid Volume Deficit

   Risk for Impaired Skin Integrity

   Risk for Injury

Nursing Management of the Newborn with Respiratory Distress

Key Points

- All preterm newborns are at risk for RDS, whether they are AGA, SGA, or LGA. Birthweight alone is not an indicator of fetal lung maturity. Gestational age, intra-uterine stress, exogenous steroid use, and ruptured membranes are among the factors that can accelerate lung maturation.

- Lack of surfactant causes alveolar instability; this increases atelectasis and leads to hypoxia and acidosis.

- Classic symptoms are sternal and intercostal retractions, flaring nares, and expiratory grunting.

- Goals of care are to:
  - Maintain adequate oxygenation and ventilation.
  - Correct acid-base imbalance.
  - Support and maintain homeostasis.

- The nurse supports homeostasis by preventing cold stress, providing adequate nutrition, and preventing infection.

- **Key Terms/Concepts**: Respiratory distress syndrome, surfactant, alveoli, dyspnea, cyanosis, sternal retractions, tachypnea, L/S ratio

Overview

Respiratory distress is a condition of the newborn marked by dyspnea, cyanosis, nasal flaring, expiratory grunting, and substernal or intercostal retractions. Respiratory distress is the major cause of death in the neonatal age group, and if the child survives, there is a high risk for chronic neurological complications. Respiratory distress syndrome (RDS) occurs primarily in premature infants, whose lungs lack adequate surfactant to maintain air sack inflation. Without surfactant, the alveoli collapse and cannot exchange oxygen and carbon dioxide. The extra work demanded by the respiratory effort can quickly deplete the newborn's energy. RDS occurs more frequently in premature Caucasian infants than in African-American infants, and about twice as often in males than in females.

Risk Factors

- Prematurity—regardless of whether the infant is appropriate, small, or large for gestational age
- Infants of diabetic mothers
- Cesarean birth
- Cardiac or pulmonary anomalies
- Precipitous delivery

Signs and Symptoms

- Low Apgar ratings at birth
- Increasing respiratory difficulty in the first three to six hours of life
- Tachypnea (>60 breaths per minute)
- Increased work of breathing: grunting, flaring nares, and retractions (subcostal, intercostal, sternal, and supraclavicular)
- Pallor
- Cyanosis: Blue discoloration of the genitalia, nailbed, lips, mouth, extremities, face, and trunk
- Apneic episodes of more than 20 seconds in duration
- Hypotonic muscle tone

Diagnostic Tests and Lab

- L/S ratio (during pregnancy): Amniotic fluid testing to show lung maturity (lecithin/ sphingomyelin). A ratio of less than 2:1 indicates immature lungs.
- Arterial blood gas determinations
- Pulse oximetry
- X-rays
- Echocardiography

Therapeutic Nursing Management

- Assist with the administration of synthetic surfactant at birth through endotracheal tube. Surfactant should be warmed to room temperature. The 4 mL/kg dosage may need to be divided into smaller aliquots and delivered with infant position changes.
- Provide humidified oxygenation for mild cases of RDS.
- Provide continuous positive airway pressure (CPAP) for moderately severe cases.
- Provide mechanical ventilation for severe cases.
- Maintain adequate hydration (usually 80-160 cc/kg/day).
- Suspend bottle feedings during periods of tachypnea to decrease the risk of aspiration.
- Maintain a thermal neutral environment and proper acid/base balance.
- Handle newborn gently and provide for rest.
- Position with the head up.
- Assess respiratory rate and effort.
- Assess skin perfusion and color.

Complications

- Atelectasis
- Persistent pulmonary hypertension
- Bronchopulmonary dysplasia

- Patent ductus arteriosus
- Acidosis
- Hypoxia
- Apnea
- Pneumothorax
- Death

Critical Thinking Exercise: Nursing Management of the Newborn with Respiratory Distress

Situation: J.B. is a premature, appropriate-for-gestational-age (AGA), male infant, who weighed 2 kg (4.4 lbs.) at birth. His Apgar scores were 5 and 7. J.B. is in an incubator, receiving oxygen and CPAP. He is attached to a cardiac monitor and a pulse oximeter. His respiratory rate is 68 per minute, heart rate is 150 beats per minute, and temperature is 97.4° F rectally. He has sternal retractions, nasal flaring, and expiratory grunting with his breathing. His mother wishes to breastfeed him, but he is presently being gavage fed because he is too lethargic to latch on and suck effectively.

1. List the client data in the situation.

2. Place an "**R**" beside the data that represent **risk** factors for RDS. Place an "**S**" beside the data that represent **symptoms** of RDS. Place an "**N**" in the blank if it is **neither** a risk factor nor a symptom of RDS.

   _____ Prematurity

   _____ AGA

   _____ Male

   _____ Apgars of 5 and 7

   _____ Respirations 68/minute

   _____ African-American

   _____ Sternal retractions, grunting, nasal flaring

   _____ Rectal temperature 97.4° F

   _____ Heart rate 150 bpm

3. What is the relationship between J.B.'s being in the incubator and his RDS?

4. Write three nursing diagnoses that would be appropriate for J.B. State both problem and etiology.

   a.

   b.

   c.

Nursing Management of the Newborn with Sepsis

Key Points

- Infants are susceptible to microorganisms that would not be harmful to older children.
- Signs of sepsis neonatorum are subtle and may resemble other diseases; the nurse most often notices them during routine care of the infant.
- Classic symptoms include: lethargy, irritability, pallor, temperature instability (usually hypothermia), feeding intolerance, jaundice, and tachycardia.
- Fever is not typically a symptom of infection in the newborn.
- Strict hand washing is essential.
- Nursing care includes antibiotic therapy and supportive care (e.g., prevent cold stress, provide respiratory and cardiovascular support, provide fluids and calories, monitor for complications).
- **Key Terms/Concepts:** Temperature instability, TORCH, GBS

Overview

Newborns are susceptible to infection by organisms that do not cause significant disease in older children. An infection in the newborn can spread rapidly through the bloodstream, regardless of its primary site. Sepsis rarely causes death in the mother, but it is the leading cause of fetal and neonatal morbidity and mortality. Infections may be acquired in utero, during delivery, or in the first month. Infections may be bacterial, viral, fungal, or parasitic. TORCH infections are the common causes of infection. TORCH is an acronym for: T toxoplasmosis, O other, R rubella, C cytomegalovirus (CMV), H herpes ("other" includes gonorrhea, syphilis, varicella, Hepatitis B, and human immunodeficiency virus).

The fetus may become infected during the passage through the birth canal, or because of infection related to prolonged rupture of membranes. Newborns may become infected from the mother, caregivers, blood transfusion equipment, or through the environment. The effects of an infection on the neonate depend on the specific infectious organism and the gestational stage at which it was acquired.

Risk Factors

- Prematurity
- Prolonged rupture of membranes (after 24 hours)
- Low socioeconomic status
- Lack of prenatal care

- Maternal substance abuse
- Low birth weight
- Multiple gestations
- Maternal infection during pregnancy, delivery, or postpartum
- Intrauterine growth retardation (IUGR)
- Nosocomial transmission after delivery
- Neonatal invasive procedures
- Maternal invasive procedures
- Maternal smoking
- Amnionitis
- Maternal bleeding
- Congenital anomalies (spina bifida, etc.)

Signs and Symptoms

- Poor feeding (decreased intake, poor suck)
- Vomiting
- Diarrhea
- Lethargy
- Cyanosis or jaundice
- Hypothermia or hyperthermia
- Full, bulging fontanels
- Jitteriness, tremors
- Seizures
- Rash
- Apnea
- Tachypnea
- Nasal flaring, grunting or retractions
- Mottling
- Pallor
- Petechiae
- Neutropenia (CSP)

Diagnostic Tests and Lab

- Cultures of blood, cerebrospinal fluid, urine, gastric aspirate
- CBC: 1:T ratio (immature: total); decreased absolute neutrophil count (ANC)
- Chest x-rays
- Blood glucose
- CSF analysis: CBC, glucose, protein
- Sediment rate

Therapeutic Nursing Management

- Isolate infected newborns.
- Administer antibiotics as ordered. Alternatively, teach parents about neonatal home infusion of antibiotics.
- Nursing care includes maintaining isolation/sterile technique and strict hand washing.
- Maintain skin integrity; assess color, appetite, stools, and temperature.
- Observe respiratory status.
- Assess for evidence of worsening condition (neutropenia).
- Provide emotional support for parents (e.g., keep them informed of the newborn's prognosis and treatment).
- Promote parent-infant bonding by allowing parents to participate in daily care as tolerated.

Complications

- Apnea
- Hypoglycemia, hyperglycemia
- Acidosis
- Hyponatremia
- Hypocalcemia
- Shock
- Failure to thrive
- Death

Critical Thinking Exercise: Nursing Management of the Newborn with Sepsis

1. Which of the following newborns is/are at risk for sepsis?

    Baby A, who was born at 35 weeks gestation and was large for gestational age

    Baby B, who was born at 40 weeks gestation and was large for gestational age

    Baby C, a triplet whose mother experienced gestational diabetes

    Baby D, whose mother took medications to treat infertility before he was conceived

    Baby E, who is Rh+ and whose mother is Rh-

    Baby F, who was born at 40 weeks gestation and is small for gestational age

    Baby G, whose mother uses cocaine and experienced several weeks of bleeding from mild placental separation.

    Baby H, whose mother worked in a factory until 4 weeks before the birth

    Baby I, who will be discharged home with his mother and father, who has tuberculosis

2. In which of the following newborns should neonatal sepsis be suspected? (Temperatures are all axillary.)

    Baby A: Temperature 100° F, dry mucous membranes, minimal urinary output

    Baby B: Temperature 97° F, feeding poorly, lethargic, pale, and jittery

    Baby C: Temperature 98.4° F, nasal flaring and grunting with respirations, mottled, with periods of apnea

    Baby D: Temperature 96.8° F, jaundiced, feeding poorly

    Baby E: Temperature 98.2° F, diarrhea, vomiting, rash

3. Which, if any, of the babies in #2 can definitely be said to have sepsis?

4. Which, if any, of the babies in #2 have symptoms that should be reported?

Situation: F.J. is two days old. She is in the neonatal intensive care unit because of sepsis neonatorum. F.J. has vomiting, diarrhea and a skin rash. She has been feeding poorly and her skin turgor is poor. Her urine output is less than normal. She is receiving intravenous Ampicillin and will be tube fed to provide calories.

5. Based on these data, what nursing diagnoses can you make for F.J.?

6. What nursing actions are needed for Risk for Infection Transmission?

Nursing Management of the Newborn with Substance Withdrawal

Key Points

- Symptoms of drug withdrawal can resemble conditions such as hypoglycemia and hypocalcemia, even though glucose and calcium values are normal.
- Symptoms and effects of maternal drug abuse vary according to the drugs used; frequently this is a combination of drugs.
- Effects are present at birth and they are often long-term.
- Newborns with **fetal alcohol syndrome** are at risk for specific congenital physical defects, along with long-term complications such as: feeding problems, CNS dysfunction, mental retardation, hyperactivity, and language abnormalities.
- Newborns of mothers who abuse other drugs experience drug withdrawal, along with the risk of growth retardation, respiratory distress, jaundice, congenital anomalies, and behavioral abnormalities.
- Nursing care is aimed at reducing withdrawal symptoms and supporting respirations, temperature, and nutrition.
- **Key Terms/Concepts:** Neonatal abstinence syndrome, FAS, IUGR.

Overview

Any prenatal substance abuse can have lifelong consequences for the neonate. For example, periodic episodes of cerebral anoxia in utero, caused by repeated withdrawal of the substance, can cause permanent brain damage in the fetus. Newborns of women who abuse alcohol or drugs may be born physiologically dependent on the abused substance and suffer from withdrawal of the substance. About 50% of newborns of addicted mothers experience severe withdrawal symptoms. Nursing assessment should include observing for the most common signs of drug withdrawal in all neonates, but especially those who have a history of maternal substance abuse.

Risk Factors

Maternal abuse of alcohol, cocaine, opiates (including methadone)

Signs and Symptoms of Maternal Drug Abuse

Alcohol abuse: Newborn facial anomalies, microcephaly, developmental delays, mental retardation, fine motor dysfunction, hypotonia, failure to thrive, cardiac septal defects, limb malformations

Cocaine abuse: Intrauterine growth retardation (IUGR), prematurity, cardiac defects, irritability, inconsolable crying, high-pitched cry, gaze aversion, increased risk for sudden infant death syndrome (SIDS), poor feeding, hypersensitivity, tremors/seizures, increased non-nutritive sucking

Opiate abuse: Hyperthermia, irritability, hypertonicity, high-pitched cry, easily startled, short sleep cycles, tachypnea, increased non-nutritive sucking, poor feeding, regurgitation, diarrhea, stuffy nose, tremors, twitching, seizures, weight loss

General Signs and Symptoms of Newborn Withdrawal

In order to make early identification of newborns needing interventions, the nurse should observe all newborns, especially those with a history of maternal drug abuse, for the following:

Central nervous system: Hyperactivity, shrill cry, muscle tension, exaggerated reflexes, tremors, seizures, sneezing, hiccups, yawning, restless sleep, fever

Gastrointestinal System: vigorous but disorganized suck, vomiting, drooling, hyperactive gag reflex, hyperphagia, diarrhea, abdominal cramping, poor feeding

Respiratory system: Tachypnea, excessive secretions, stuffy nose, yawning, sneezing

Skin: Excoriations of buttocks, knees, and elbows; scratches on the face; circumoral pallor, flushing, sweating

Diagnostic Tests

- Serological test for syphilis, HIV, and hepatitis B
- Urine drug screen
- Meconium analysis

Pharmacologic Management

Medications used to control withdrawal symptoms include:

- Phenobarbital
- Paregoric
- Morphine sulfate
- Donnatal
- Simethicone (Mylicon)

Therapeutic Nursing Management

- Determine the mother's last drug intake (time and amount).
- Provide rest and adequate newborn nutrition (withdrawal requires expenditure of energy).
- Provide small, frequent feedings; intravenous therapy if needed.
- Monitor pulse and respirations every 15 minutes until stable; stimulate if apnea occurs.
- Observe for difficulty adjusting to environmental stimuli, such as noises and bright lights. Place in quiet area with dim lights.
- Reduce neonatal stimulation.
- Swaddle infant snugly.
- Use calming techniques and rocking.

- Position on right side to prevent aspiration of vomitus and secretions.
- Administer gastric hypermotility medications as ordered.
- Maintain skin integrity.
- Assess seizure activity.
- Assess respiratory effectiveness.
- Evaluate parenting behaviors.
- Refer for home care as appropriate.
- Refer to social service for support.

Complications

- Congenital anomalies
- Seizures
- Long-term behavioral and attachment problems
- Sudden infant death syndrome (SIDS)

Critical Thinking Exercise: Nursing Management of the Newborn with Substance Withdrawal

Situation: B.J. is 72 hours old. He was born prematurely at 32 weeks' gestation and was exposed to cocaine and heroin in utero. He is SGA, not feeding well, but sucks frantically on a pacifier. He is being fed through a nasogastric tube and regurgitates much of his feedings. His temperature is 100° F, pulse is 140, and respirations are 70 per minute. He is on an apnea monitor. B. J. has had six watery stools in the past 24 hours and has lost 10% of his birth weight. He has mild tremors when stimulated, and cries often with a high-pitched cry.

1. What symptoms of maternal cocaine abuse does B.J. have?

2. What symptoms of maternal opiate abuse does B.J. have?

3. For which complications should the nurse be especially watchful?

4. What would be important to include in teaching with B.J. mother/parent?

5. Why is it important to refer B.J.'s family to social services? What other community resources would be critical for this family?

Critical Thinking Exercise Answer Keys

Situation: Keysha and her partner, Kevin, are native Americans expecting their first baby's birth in approximately 8 weeks. They have come to the pre-admission clinic to discuss their plans for labor and birth. As the nurse in the clinic, you describe and discuss some of the options for labor and birth that are available to them. It is their wish to have several family members present at the time of birth and to burn sweet grass during labor.

Using the concepts of family-centered care, connect with arrows or lines the care planning and interventions that the nurse may include to the correct concept(s) of family-centered care (more than one may apply).

Concept	Care Planning and Interventions
Choice	Discuss choices for labor regarding pain management and people present.
Collaboration	Prepare the birthing unit staff for their request, determine any safety and fire precautions that need to be put in place.
Empowerment	Encourage this family to continue with their traditions by the use of their sweet grass ceremony at birth.
Flexibility	Encourage this couple to think about all of their options and to be comfortable choosing different ones depending on how they work in labor.
Information	Provide information about the hospital's birthing unit, number of family members encouraged to be present, how others might be accommodated and how their wishes regarding birth may be accommodated.
Respect	Involve this couple in the birth planning by documenting their wishes and communicating them to the birthing unit staff.
Strengths	Encourage this family to build on their support system by doing their ceremony at birth, having family members present and including them when teaching is done.
Support	Discuss the role of the support person with this couple and provide information on what might be helpful in labour.

Health promotion regarding postpartum depression is a current focus in maternal/child nursing as a result of research that has shown that the incidence is much higher than was previously thought. The time that a postpartum woman and her family spend in the hospital is very short. How and when might you teach about postpartum depression to ensure that each woman and her family have enough information about this important health concern?

---

1. When?

  • Prenatally in childbirth education classes
  • Pre-admission clinic for her hospital stay
  • Postpartum teaching in hospital
  • Community clinics for well baby/mothers afterwards

2. How?

  • With other family members present so that they receive information as well

3. What adult learning principles would be utilized with this teaching plan?

  • Repetition
  • Teachable moments
  • Follow-up
  • Presenting material in different formats and offering amounts

4. How would you evaluate your teaching with a family?

- **Ask them to repeat it back to you or describe it to you in their own words.**
- **Ask them to tell you about their specific community resources and how they would contact them.**

5. What if a couple or woman/family member had a language barrier, e.g. first language is Spanish?

- **Ensure that there is an interpreter present for the teaching.**
- **Include resources that are written in the woman's language if possible.**

Critical Thinking Exercise: CHAPTER 3

Medication Administration Answer Key

1. Ms. S., a G3 TPAL 2002 woman, has indicated in a birth plan that she hopes to use comfort measures during her labor and birth. However, the physician has determined that she needs augmentation for her labor based on her lack of progress. What information would you include in describing the potential side effects and benefits of Oxytocin to augment labor?

   Answers would include:
   - **Benefit of decreased waiting for labor to increase and birth to occur, side effects may include decreased mobility (need to monitor contractions continuously and fetal heart rate SOGC guidelines)**
   - **Contractions will increase in strength and frequency more quickly than normal labor due to Oxytocin (may increase woman's need for pain medication).**

2. She finds the contractions to be frequent and strong and requests information about an epidural. She is 4 cm dilated, 100% effaced and is thinking that it might be helpful. What risks and benefits would you describe to Ms. S.?

   Answers would include:
   - **Benefit to pain relief**
   - **Side effects/risks include decreased mobility**
   - **Potential for risks related to insertion and medication**

3. Her labor progresses rapidly once the Oxytocin has been started and an epidural is inserted. Post birth, she has strong after-pains when her baby is breastfeeding. What information would you provide Ms. S. for pain relief (include pharmacologic strategies as well as comfort measures)?

   Answers would include:
   - **Ibuprofen as the pharmacological strategy (best drug due to anti-inflammatory properties as well as analgesia)**
   - **Taking medication prior to breastfeeding**
   - **Breastfeeding positions that do not involve resting the baby on the abdomen**
   - **Information about usual length of time they last**

Situation: A teenage girl, age 15, says that her periods are "really bad." She says, "They're so unpredictable sometimes every 24-25 days, sometimes every 32 days. They are heavy, too. I use five or six tampons a day, and I usually have cramps and pain, particularly on the first day. Is this normal?"

1. What should the nurse tell her? What self-care measures should she suggest?

   The flow she is describing is quite normal. It is common for teenagers to have irregular cycles. The cramps, too, are normal, and indicate that she is having ovulatory cycles. The nurse should reassure her that there is nothing wrong. The nurse could suggest that she take a prostaglandin inhibitor (e.g., ibuprofen) for cramping. A hot tub, a heating pad, warm tea, or any other source of warmth may ease the cramping. Daily aerobic exercise (e.g., swimming, walking) can also help to prevent cramps and other menstrual difficulties. Good nutrition is also important.

2. The girl says, "I don't see how heat would help the cramps. What does it do?" What should the nurse tell her?

   Tell her that heat, in general, is soothing. In addition, it increases blood flow to the abdomen and promotes relaxation.

Situation: A woman tells the nurse that she plans to use natural family planning (no contraceptives). She says that she knows how to recognize that ovulation has occurred. The nurse asks for clarity and the woman states that she has an increase in vaginal discharge in the middle of her cycle and that the mucous is "thin and slippery" at this time.

1. Is this a normal sign of ovulation?

    Yes, this clear, slippery mucous is produced mid-cycle to aid in sperm motility into the uterus.

2. What other signs of ovulation could the woman be taught if she wishes to use natural family planning?

    Temperature taking and charting to see increase in temperature with ovulation, and accurate documentation of menses and cycle to track patterns to anticipate ovulation.

Situation: A newly pregnant woman remarks, "My mother says I have to eat lots of meat if I want this baby to be a boy. Do you know of anything else that I can do to help? My husband says he does not want a wife who cannot give him sons, and I'm afraid to disappoint him."

3. How accurate is this woman's understanding of reproductive physiology? What information does she need before she can begin coping and making informed decisions about her situation?

    The pregnant woman clearly does not understand that the sex of her baby is determined by the chromosomes. Certainly, dietary intake has no bearing on increasing the likelihood of conceiving a child of a particular gender. The nurse's plan for this woman's prenatal care should include teaching pertaining to: (a) the sex of the baby is determined at fertilization, and (b) the sperm containing X and Y chromosomal material determines the baby's sex. In addition, it is obvious there are emotional, relational, and other issues this woman is

dealing with at this time. The nurse should use active listening and other therapeutic communication techniques to help the woman explore her own feelings and cope with the news of her pregnancy. However, there could be other significant interpersonal or sociocultural factors coming into play that are beyond the scope of this section of the review.

Critical Thinking Exercise: CHAPTER 6

Fetal Development Answer Key

Situation: J.M. is in her third trimester of pregnancy. She has been given ampicillin for a kidney infection, and is very worried about the possible effects on the fetus. She says, "What if it causes a defect in the baby's heart, or kidneys, or something?"

---

1. Without even knowing anything specific about the medication J.M. is taking, how realistic are her fears? What can the nurse tell her about fetal development that may help to decrease her fears?

> Most organ formation takes place during weeks 3-8 of gestation (the embryonic period). The third trimester is a time during which the fetus matures and gains weight; it is not a critical time for teratogenic effects. Although pregnant women should always check with their primary care provider before taking any medications, they are less likely to be harmful this late in pregnancy.

Situation: M.P. has come to the clinic on September 10th. She states that the first day of her last menstrual period was June 10. She has performed a home pregnancy test, which was positive. She says, "I think that I may be pregnant. I've had nausea in the morning and vomiting (2-3 times/week). M.P. tells you as the nurse in the clinic that she had an abortion when she was 18. She also had a miscarriage at 11 weeks last year. On examination, Chadwick and Hegar's signs are present. M.P. states that she is often tired and that for the past three months, she has experienced urinary frequency.

1. From this data, can you be sure that M.P. is pregnant? Why or why not?

   No, you cannot be sure. None of the positive signs of pregnancy are present. All signs are either presumptive or probable–that is, they could be caused by something other than pregnancy.

2. What information do you need to confirm M.P.'s pregnancy?

   Either auscultation of fetal heart tones, palpation of fetal movement by an examiner (not M.P.), and/or visualization of the fetus on sonogram

3. What information would you give M.P. regarding nausea and vomiting during pregnancy?

   None. All are normal changes of pregnancy.

4. What is M.P.'s due date, or estimated date of birth (EDB)?

> **LMP = June 10**
>
> **Subtract 3 months = March 10**
>
> **Add 7 days**
>
> **EDC = March 17**

5. Using the terms, "gravida" and "para" and the TPAL method for describing obstetrical history, describe M.P.'s GTAL. (gravida 3, para 0, TPAL: 30020)

As a gravida 4, para 3, multipara, or a multigravida. The term "primi-" would not be applicable for her.

Situation: C.J. is at the end of the first trimester of her pregnancy. Her normal prepregnant weight was 120 lbs. She now weighs 125 lbs, and she is concerned that she is "getting fat." Her food diary indicates that she is eating a fairly well balanced diet except for an insufficient intake of dairy products and iron-rich foods. She says, "I don't drink milk. I've never liked it." C.J. states that she has been taking her folic acid supplement as prescribed.

---

1. How would you assess C.J.'s weight gain: too much, too little, or just right?

   An "average" gain in first trimester is 3.5 lbs. She has gained a little more than that, but certainly not enough to be concerned about from a health standpoint.

2. With regard to C.J.'s weight, what problem should be of most concern to the nurse?

   Because C.J. sees herself as fat, she may decrease her calorie intake. This could have negative consequences for both her and the fetus.

3. How should the nurse respond to C.J.'s statement that she doesn't like milk?

   The nurse should teach her the importance of dairy products in providing calcium and protein needed for fetal development, and about other dairy products that she can substitute for milk (cheese, cottage cheese, yogurt, custard puddings, and ice cream). If these are not acceptable to C.J., then other sources of protein (meat, eggs) must be found; and a calcium supplement may be necessary.

4. What medical complication is likely to occur if C.J.'s iron intake remains low?

   Anemia

5. C.J's caregiver prescribes an iron supplement. Why do you think this was necessary? Why didn't the nurse simply advise her to eat more iron-rich foods, in the same way she addressed her dairy products deficiency?

It is almost impossible to eat enough iron-rich foods to supply the additional amount of iron needed during pregnancy.

6. How would it further complicate C.J.'s nutritional status if she were a strict vegetarian?

C.J.'s diet may already be deficient in protein and iron because of her present diet. A vegetarian diet would mean that she couldn't get protein and iron from meat and eggs.

7. How would it further complicate her nutritional status if she were a smoker?

She might be even more iron deficient. Smoking decreases the ability to absorb vitamin C; vitamin C is necessary for iron absorption.

C.J. asks specific questions to ensure that she is eating to get enough calories and nutritive value. For each of the nutrients listed below, choose two foods and the correct amount that should be in the diet of a pregnant woman:

Nutrient			Amount	Foods
Calcium	2	13	1. 15mg	8. brown bread, beef
Folic Acid	5	12	2. 1300mg	9. broccoli, strawberries
Iron	3	14	3. 30mg	10. eggs, cheese
Protein	4	10	4. 60g	11. fortified margarine, fruits
Vitamin A	7	11	5. 600ug	12. oranges, asparagus
Vitamin C	6	9	6. 70mg	13. spinach, baked beans
Zinc	1	8	7. 800ug	14. spinach, dried fruits

Situation: A pregnant woman comes to the the clinic for her regular 24 week appointment and reports some symptoms she is having. She says that she is having urinary frequency, but no burning with urination; and that her temperature is 99.1° F. She also reports that she is having a mucoid discharge from her vagina.

1. What additional assessments and history taking will the nurse do?

   What is frequency, color of urine, amount of fluid intake, overall signs and symptoms of wellness, any other symptoms of illness/infection other than fever, any bleeding from the vagina. Just to be sure, the nurse should collect a urine sample and dip for leukocytes, protein and glucose (send for culture and sensitivity if leukocytes present).

2. What else does the nurse need to know in order to be certain that the woman's vaginal discharge is normal?

   What color is it? Is it clear or cloudy? Is there any blood in it? What does it smell like? How much is there?

3. This same woman returns at 28 weeks. What would be included in her teaching at this time? List 3 topics and at least two things that would be taught to ensure that this woman knows what to do in these situations.

   Fetal movement count: If the woman is not able to count at least 10 movements over a two-hour period twice a day, then the nurse would advise her to seek immediate obstetric care.

   Preterm Labor: Cramping or backache that comes and goes and is occurring every 10-15 minutes, increasing in intensity. Notify care provider or come to the Birthing Area Triage area.

   Vaginal discharge (rupture of membranes or bleeding): Any increase in fluid from the vagina that does not stop with contraction of the muscles or any bleeding should be reported to the care provider immediately.

Situation: K.L. has been admitted to the hospital with a diagnosis of hyperemesis gravidarum. She is in the ninth week of her pregnancy and has lost 5% of her prepregnant weight. She cannot tolerate oral fluids or food, and she is receiving lactated Ringer's solution intravenously (IV).

1. What nursing diagnoses would be appropriate for K.L.?

    Risk for Fluid Volume Deficit (She probably has Actual Fluid Volume Deficit; however, there is not enough information in this situation to be sure of that.)

    Altered Nutrition: Less than Body Requirements/ Nausea/Fear (related to fetal well-being)

2. All of the data suggest that K.L. is at risk for Altered Nutrition. Which data specifically supports a diagnosis of actual Altered Nutrition?

    The facts indicate that she has lost 5% of her prepregnant weight.

3. Why is K.L. receiving intravenous fluids?

    She is receiving intravenous fluids to prevent or treat dehydration.

K.L. continues to be very nauseous and vomits 3-4 times a day. The gastroenterologist involved in her care recommends total parenteral nutrition (TPN) until she is able to keep oral intake down. She and her husband receive training in preparation for home care. She tells you that she is worried about the next few weeks and has even considered terminating the pregnancy.

4. As her nurse, you tell her to:?

    a.   Focus on the baby and the nausea will gradually decrease.

    b.   Use guided imagery to take her to a safe place and try to relax.

    c.   Talk about her feelings whenever she wants and that they are normal.

    d.   Focus on her discharge home and that once home she will probably feel better.

5. What other professionals would you consider involving in K.L.'s care prior to discharge?

    Social worker

    Pastoral care

    Physiotherapist (to address bedrest)

Situation: S.J. is a 38-year-old primigravida at 32 weeks gestation. She lives with her parents and t
sisters. She has a high-stress sales job being paid by commissions only. She admits that she doesn't
right." She says she doesn't have time to prepare meals and eats mostly fast foods and "junk food." H
mother does cook for the family, but the meals are high in fat and sodium. S.J. is 5 ft. 2 in. tall and he
prepregnant weight was 180 lbs. S.J. has edema of the feet, ankles, and hands.

1. What risk factors does S.J. have for pregnancy-induced hypertension?

   **She is older than 35, has a poor diet, has a stressful job, is overweight, and this is her first
   pregnancy.**

2. What vital sign is the most important for the nurse to assess at this time?

   Blood pressure

3. What should the nurse ask S.J. in order to assess her edema further?

   **Ask her if it improves after she has been in bed; that is, is the edema less first thing in the
   morning and worse at the end of the day?**

wo
eat
er

9. Her health problem will be managed on an outpatient basis. After
 d pressure and to check her urine for protein, she is asked to keep a
 in, B/P, and fetal movement count. What other advice should the

 g her prenatal appointments.

 f her symptoms worsen.

 rictions.

 ed for good nutrition, especially protein.

 S.J. the signs of worsening preeclampsia and advise her to telephone immediately if
 any of the signs occur (e.g., B/P increase to 160/110, facial edema, decreased urine output,
increased proteinuria, headaches, epigastric pain, nausea and vomiting).

Situation: K.C. is 34 years old. She is a gravida 2, para 0. Her first pregnancy ended in a stillbirth. At her first prenatal visit her diabetes screening was negative. However, in her second trimester, she is diagnosed with gestational diabetes. She is normal weight for her height, and her weight gain has followed the recommended pattern thus far in pregnancy.

1. What risk factors does K.C. have for gestational diabetes?

   She is older than 30 and has a history of fetal demise.

2. What test was probably used to diagnose K.C.'s diabetes?

   An oral glucose tolerance test, probably a 3-hour test, administered after an overnight fast

3. Why do you think K.C.'s urine was negative for glucose on her first prenatal visit, but her glucose screening test was positive during her second trimester?

   Fetal nutrient demands rise during the second trimester, requiring the mother to increase her calorie intake. This creates greater blood glucose levels. At the same time, the woman becomes resistant to insulin because of the insulin antagonistic effects of the placental hormones, cortisol, and insulinase. Maternal insulin demands rise dramatically at this time. Most women can produce enough insulin to compensate for their insulin resistance; however, some cannot, so gestational diabetes results. About half the women who develop gestational diabetes will become diabetic later in life.

4. K.C.'s glucose tolerance test was initially >95 mg/dL (>5.3 mmol/L) and her 1 hour test was >180 mg/dL (>10.0 mmol/L). How would you interpret these results? How would you plan her care?

> The medical diagnosis of gestational diabetes will be assigned.

> The nurse will obtain a nutritional consultation for education about ADA dietary recommendations.

> The nurse will educate the pregnant woman about the importance of consistent, antepartum care because of the increased risk for fetal loss during pregnancy.

> The nurse will educate the pregnant woman about the importance of consistent, antepartum care because of the risks to the developing fetus. The first trimester of pregnancy is most critical for stable glucose control in order to reduce the chance of congenital anomalies in infants born to women with gestational diabetes.

> Additionally, the neonates are more prone to hypoglycemia, respiratory distress syndrome, hypocalcemia, and hyperbilirubinemia. Glucose management is a critical aspect of the care of the pregnancy and must be monitored diligently.

5. During labor her blood glucose levels may need to be monitored every 1-2 hours. How would you explain this?

> It is important to closely monitor the blood glucose levels because of the increased metabolic needs during labor; therefore, the woman is at risk for glucose intolerance or hypoglycemia. Additionally, dietary intake is reduced or the client may be receiving IV solution during labor.

6. K.C. has decided to breastfeed this baby. How would you encourage her with this process?

> The nurse would provide information regarding benefits of breastfeeding including: 1) maintaining a stable blood sugar in the infant, 2) promotion of maternal-infant attachment, 3) passing an immununologic benefit to the infant, and 4) aiding in maternal weight loss (approximately 500 Kcal/day for the average woman) .

Situation: T.C. is in the 26th week of her pregnancy. Her hemoglobin is 9.5 g/dL and her hematocrit is 30%. She says, "My sister's hemoglobin was low, too. They said it was normal, though, because your blood is 'thinner' during pregnancy. I'm glad I'm not anemic."

1. How should the nurse respond to T.C.'s statement?

   When a pregnant woman's hemoglobin is slightly low, this may, indeed be due to hemodilution (the blood plasma volume increases more than the red blood cell mass). However, T.C.'s hemoglobin and hematocrit are below the lower limits of the normal range; she is anemic.

2. The care provider prescribes an oral iron supplement for T.C. The nurse tells her that she should include foods high in vitamin C (e.g., oranges, grapefruits, tomatoes, melons, and strawberries). Why?

   Vitamin C increases the absorption of the iron supplement.

3. The nurse also tells T.C. to avoid consuming these foods at the same time as taking the iron supplement: bran, egg yolk, oxalates (e.g., spinach), coffee, tea, and milk. She advises her to take her iron supplement between meals. Why?

   These foods decrease iron absorption; iron is best absorbed on an empty stomach.

4. One week later, T.C. telephones to say that she has abdominal discomfort after taking her iron pill. What should the nurse advise?

   T.C. might try taking the pill at bedtime. If this does not help, then she might eat a small amount of food (e.g., a cracker) when taking the pill.

5. During this same telephone call, T.C. tells the nurse that she is not constipated, but that her stools are black. What should the nurse advise?

Tell T.C. that this is a normal side effect of iron supplements.

Situation: A woman in the 14th week of pregnancy is admitted with a dilated cervix, severe abdominal cramping, and heavy vaginal bleeding. She is diagnosed with inevitable miscarriage (abortion).

---

1. What should the initial nursing assessment include- and why?

   The nurse should collect data about:
   - **Pain: To determine appropriate interventions for pain**
   - **Amount of bleeding: For early detection and treatment of hemorrhage**
   - **Temperature: To determine whether infection is present and to provide a baseline if it is not**
   - **Pulse and blood pressure: As indicators of hemorrhage and to provide a baseline**
   - **Emotional status: The parents are commonly anxious and fearful regarding what may happen to the woman and the fetus.**
   - **Previous pregnancies and previous pregnancy losses: These may provide insight into emotional status.**
   - **Allergies: Because medications may need to be given**

2. Based on the data provided in the situation, what nursing diagnoses can you be sure this woman has? (Write the etiologies of the diagnoses, as well.)

   Pain related to uterine contractions

   Risk for fluid volume deficit related to heavy bleeding

   Risk for infection related to dilated cervix

3. For what other nursing diagnoses should the nurse assess?

   Anxiety/fear related to unknown outcome and unfamiliarity with procedures/treatments

Anticipatory grieving related to unexpected outcome of pregnancy

Situational low self-esteem related to inability to carry the pregnancy to term

4. What expected outcomes are appropriate for this woman?

- Reports relief from pain
- Experiences no signs or symptoms of hemorrhage or infection (e.g., vital signs within normal limits, no excessive bleeding)
- Discusses the impact of the loss on her and her family
- Expresses understanding that she did nothing to cause the miscarriage

5. This woman has experienced or is experiencing a loss. How would you incorporate her partner's emotional needs in her care planning while at the hospital/clinic? What follow-up would be appropriate for this woman/partner?

Provide choices where she is to stay, express your sympathy, provide information as requested and regarding physical signs and symptoms that will be normal when going home.

Appropriate follow-up should include referral to bereavement support groups if available and public health for follow-up.

Situation: A.J. has just given birth. She will go home 48 hours after the delivery. She is breastfeeding her baby. Her antepartum rubella titer was 1:8.

1. Should she receive rubella vaccine before leaving the hospital? Why or why not?

   Yes. Her titer indicates that she is serologically not immune. She should be immunized to prevent a rubella infection during future pregnancies.

2. What questions should the nurse ask A.J. to determine if the rubella vaccine is contraindicated for her? Why?

   Ask if she is allergic to eggs. If the vaccine is made from duck eggs, she may develop a hypersensitivity reaction if she is allergic to eggs.

   Ask if she or any other household members are immunocompromised because the virus is shed in urine and other body fluids.

3. What should the nurse teach A.J. about the vaccine?

   She can continue to breastfeed because the live attenuated virus is not communicable.

   She may have a rash and transient arthritis;both are benign.

   She must practice contraception to avoid pregnancy for one month after being vaccinated.

   She might expect side effects to occur within 10-14 days after the vaccine is given. The nurse educates the postpartum woman about pregnancy prevention measures for at least one month after the rH immune globulin is administered. Follow-up serum blood level is needed to determine the immunity prior to future

   pregnancy.

Situation: Elaine, a woman at 33 weeks of gestation is admitted to the hospital with a diagnosis of placenta previa. She is not in labor and is having only mild vaginal bleeding and spotting. Her fetal heart rate is within normal limits for rate and pattern. She is receiving "expectant management" (that is, observation and bed rest) rather than being immediately scheduled for a cesarean birth. Medical orders include the following:

1. Her medical orders appear on the left side of the chart. Write the rationale for these orders and the health teaching that would be included with each one.

Medical Order	Rationale	Teaching
Weekly biophysical profile	Assessment of fetal growth and development	Describe normal fetal growth and development weekly
Daily NST	Ongoing assessment of fetal growth	Explanation of fetal heart rate, variability and accelerations (and significance)
Weekly CBC	Assess for bleeding (internal)	Need for ongoing assessment
Physiotherapy consult	Bedrest includes decreased mobility and risk for DVT and muscle wasting.	Describe need for exercise, even on bedrest
Nutritional consult	Need for diet to be appropriate to pregnancy	Nutrional requirements of pregnancy
Vital signs q6h (BP, P and FHR)	Ongoing assessment (maternal and fetal)	Understanding the need of assessment
Venous access device	Ability to access IV for fluids/ blood if needed ASAP	Understanding of condition and treatment
Betamethasone 12 mg IM stat and then repeat in 12 hours	Fetal Lung development	Understanding of medication and its effect

2. Elaine has a 2-year-old at home and a husband who works shift-work. Being on bedrest is a hardship for her for care of her child at home. How would you offer assistance with this?

Community resources, discussion of family who might help, and assistance with phone or internet (computer access) to be in touch with daughter/husband

Situation: A woman at 35 weeks of gestation is admitted to the hospital with a small amount of vaginal bleeding and moderately severe abdominal pain. The fetal heart rate is within normal limits for rate and pattern. Her blood pressure has been elevated for the past month, and is 160/90 today. Her pulse is 80, temperature is 98.6° F, and respirations are 14. The nursing history reveals that she is underweight and does not maintain a healthy diet. She says, "I don't know how I can stand to stay here if you don't let me smoke." Medical orders include the following:

- Continuous electronic fetal monitoring
- Indwelling urinary catheter
- Intravenous fluids
- Give betamethasone (a glucocorticoid) 12 mg intramuscular q12hrs x two doses

1. What are the risk factors that may have contributed to this woman's placental abruption?

   Elevated blood pressure, smoking, and poor nutrition

2. Why was an indwelling urinary catheter ordered?

   It is the best way to evaluate fluid volume and maternal organ perfusion.

3. Why were intravenous fluids ordered?

   To maintain fluid volume, and as a route for administering blood and other blood products (e.g., frozen plasma may be needed to maintain the fibrinogen level)

4. While you are assisting her to her birthing room, reviewing her obstetrical history and vital signs, you observe her increasing distress with pain. Your abdominal palpation suggests that her abdomen is becoming more taut and tender. The fetal heart rate baseline has decreased from 120 bpm to 108 bpm. What is your plan of care for this woman/family?

Ensure that she has blood cross-matched for emergency, notify the care provider, increase of IV fluid and continue to monitor her vital signs and FHR.

5. How would you describe your plan of care to this woman/family?

Describe the steps you are taking and that you will stay with her and continue to keep her informed.

6. What is the most logical explanation for what is happening?

Placental abruption

Situation: At her first prenatal visit, a woman says, "My friend had TORCH infection when she was pregnant, and her baby died. Can I get an immunization to prevent that disease?"

1. How should the nurse answer this question?

   Explain that it is not a single disease, but several separate diseases, mainly viruses. There are no vaccinations for most of them, except for rubella and hepatitis B. Rubella vaccine is contraindicated during pregnancy; however, she will have screening tests for the TORCH infections so that they can be properly managed if they occur. There are some measures she can take to prevent infection.

2. The woman says, "What can I do to keep from getting these infections and passing them to my baby?" What advice should the nurse give to her?

   The mother should report any influenza-like symptoms or other symptoms of infections to her health care provider. Early detection of any infection she has may make it possible to decrease the effects on the fetus. Specifically, to avoid toxoplasmosis, she should use good hand washing technique, avoid eating raw meat, and avoid exposure to cat litter. To avoid hepatitis B, she should not use contaminated needles (if she is an intravenous drug user) and she should practice "safe sex." Practicing safe sex should also prevent herpes. To help prevent rubella, she should avoid children and people who have not been vaccinated. Risks for CMV include working or having a child in a day care center, an institution for the mentally retarded, or in certain health settings (e.g., dialysis); she should avoid those situations if possible.

3. For which of the TORCH infections are immunizations available?

   Rubella and hepatitis B

Situation: An adolescent comes to the clinic for the first time when she is in the third trimester of pregnancy. She has gained only five pounds over her stated prepregnant weight. Her partner states that they have the occasional beer on the weekend.

1. How should the nurse proceed to assess this client for substance abuse?

   The nurse must remain nonjudgmental because such an attitude will interfere with the development of trust; the client would then not report her consumption accurately. A good way to begin is to ask the woman what over-the-counter and prescribed medications she uses (ask non-threatening questions before threatening ones). Then ask about her use of legal drugs, such as caffeine, nicotine, and alcohol. Finally, the nurse should ask about her use of illicit drugs (e.g., marijuana, cocaine, heroin), and document the frequency and amount of each.

2. The client admits to smoking and "drinking quite a bit of coffee" and other caffeinated beverages. She finally tells the nurse that she drinks beer, "at least one or two a day," and that she sometimes takes "speed" to wake up when she is "hung over" from drinking. Because the client is clearly using substances, what other conditions should the nurse suspect and screen for?

   Depression, low self-esteem, anxiety, and a history of, or presently existing, physical or sexual abuse

3. Why was verbal screening necessary? What does the nurse need to do to obtain a urine- screening test for substances?

   Some substances (primarily alcohol) are undetectable within a few hours after ingestion. Also, it would not be ethical to screen the client's urine without her consent.

Situation: B.K., a 15-year-old adolescent in her sixth month of pregnancy, has come to the clinic for her first prenatal visit. She lives at home with her parents, and will continue to do so after the birth of the baby. B.K. says she does not know who the baby's father is.

---

1. Because of B.K.'s age, what assessments are especially important to make?

   Nutritional status, dietary pattern, and weight gain

   Incest or sexual abuse (especially in very young adolescents)

   B.K.'s plans for returning to school after the birth of the baby

   Her understanding of the importance of continuing prenatal care

   Blood pressure (because of her increased risk of pregnancy-induced hypertension)

   Family support as this is an important consideration of the overall wellness of the family and its response to illness

2. Why is the transition to parenthood especially difficult for adolescent parents?

   The developmental tasks of parenthood are often complicated by the unmet developmental needs of adolescence (e.g., establishing one's identity). Adolescents may have difficulty adjusting to their changing self-image and roles. Peers are very important at this life stage, and the adolescent mother may feel "different" and isolated from her peers. Developmentally, adolescents are commonly egocentric in their thinking, they are impulsive and may have a low tolerance for frustration. In addition, there are often psychosocial difficulties related to interrupted education and inadequate income.

3. For what physical complications are B.K. and her baby at especially high risk?

Low birth weight baby

Pregnancy-induced hypertension

Infant abuse or abandonment

Inadequate nutrition

4. In order to promote a healthy pregnancy, what is the most important nursing intervention at this time?

Encourage continued prenatal care visits; make any referrals needed to assure that there is support for continued prenatal care.

Situation: L.L. is 20 weeks pregnant. She has signed a consent form and is having an amniocentesis so that amniotic fluid can be obtained. Her maternal serum screening test came back with a high chance of spina bifida. She has determined with her partner and genetic counselor that she would like to rule out any false positives or negatives and to know for sure if her baby will have spina bifida. After the initial ultrasonography, the nurse directs L.L. to empty her bladder before the amniocentesis is performed.

1. Why was it necessary for L.L. to empty her bladder?

   L.L. empties her bladder to decrease the risk of perforating it with the amniocentesis needle.

2. Why was ultrasonography used along with amniocentesis?

   Ultrasonography is used to visualize the placenta, the fetus, and internal organs, to minimize accidental perforation with the needle.

3. The obstetrician states that he needs to inform L.L. of the risks and benefits of this procedure. What will be included in his discussion with L.L.?

   All procedures carry at least some risk, but complications with amniocentesis are not frequent (1%, if she asks for a figure). The nurse should explain that L. L. will not have general anesthetic and that she may feel some pressure or pain for a short time when the needle is inserted through her abdomen. The nurse will monitor her for a while after the procedure to assure her safety.

4. What assessments should be made after the procedure?

   • **Monitor vital signs**
   • **Observe for bleeding or leaking of amniotic fluid at the puncture site**
   • **Monitor for pain or uterine contractions**

Contraction Stress and Non-Stress Test Monitoring Answer Key

Situation: A woman at 33 weeks of gestation is having a non-stress test. The nurse seats her comfortably in a reclining chair and places a Doppler transducer and a Tocotransducer on her abdomen. She hands the woman a hand-held device with a button on the end.

1. The woman asks, "What am I supposed to do with this button thing?" What instructions should the nurse give her?

   The device is an event marker. Ask the woman to press the button each and every time she feels fetal movement. This will make a mark on the monitor strip that can be correlated with the FHR.

2. The woman asks, "Will this take very long? I have to meet a client at 3 o'clock." What should the nurse tell her?

   The test can probably be completed in 20-30 minutes if the fetus is active. If the fetus needs to be awakened from a sleep state, it may take longer.

3. After 20 minutes, no fetal movements have occurred and no FHR accelerations have been noted. The woman says, "Are we all through now?" What should the nurse tell her?

   Not quite. Your baby hasn't been moving, so we can't really evaluate the heart pattern. The baby may be sleeping. We need to try to awaken her/him and monitor for a little longer.

4. The woman says, "My sister had a stress test and it put her into labor. I'm not even near my due date. Will that happen to me?" What should the nurse tell her?

   Tell her that this is a non-stress test, and it is very different from what her sister probably had. Her sister most likely had a CST, which uses a medication to stimulate uterine contractions. The non-stress test is completely safe and has no side effects.

5. After 10 more minutes, the monitor shows three FHR accelerations of 12 beats per minute, lasting 20 seconds each. Is this a reactive or a nonreactive test? Is that a reassuring finding, or not?

It is a reactive test; that is a reassuring finding, indicative of fetal well-being.

Case Study: The Antepartum Client

Situation: A 23-year-old client and her husband are expecting their first baby. The client thinks she is about 10 weeks pregnant, and this is her first prenatal visit. She and her husband speak fluent Spanish, but have difficulty speaking English. They have many questions and are excited about the baby. All laboratory tests and the physical exam are within normal limits. The nurse plans to begin some antepartum teaching during this clinic visit.

Instructions: With a partner, list the danger signs of pregnancy that you will teach the client and her husband. Identify two ways you can teach the information.

DANGER SIGNS	TEACHING METHODS
1. Report vaginal bleeding or leakage - note color and time.	1. Assess the client's understanding of normal physiological changes.
2. Report bloody urine, painful urination, or decreased urinary output.	2. Use pamphlets and posters written in Spanish.
3. Report weight gain of more than 5 pounds since last prenatal visit; swelling of face, fingers; headache; dizziness; blurred vision; epigastric pain.	3. Use Spanish audio-visual materials in the clinic and for check out to client's home.
	4. Review danger signs at next client visit.
4. Check body temperature if feeling hot or flushed. Report fever greater than 101° F.	5. Teach family to use "kick sheet" for fetal activity at 20 weeks.
5. Report vomiting persisting more than 1 day.	6. Explore possibility of anyone in the home speaking English; request them to come to the next visit.
6. Report decrease in fetal activity or lack of movement for more than 6 hours.	7. One-to-one teaching via lecture/ discussion: will need an interpreter.
7. Report low backache and uterine tightening before 36 weeks gestation.	

The client returns for her 16-week checkup to the clinic. Her vital signs are 118/80, pulse 80, respirations 16. Her urine studies are normal, but her hemoglobin is 11.0 gm/dL and hematocrit is 32%. Which foods should the nurse advise the client to eat?

Since the client is anemic, foods rich in iron should be eaten. Cultural issues should be included in the diet plan (in Spanish cultures, illness and physiological conditions are either "hot" or "cold," and eating foods of the opposite category will bring back a balance to the body).

Foods include: beef, corn and vegetables, fruits such as apricots

At the next clinic visit, the client is scheduled to have a routine ultrasound of her fetus. What will you do to prepare her for the event?

Instructions: Write a paragraph or two detailing the instructions and information you would give the client about the ultrasonography.

During your next clinic visit, you are going to have a test called an ultrasound. The purpose of this test is to assess your baby's overall health, age, growth, and development. This is a painless procedure, which will not cause any problems for you or the baby. It will take about 20-30 minutes.

You will probably need a full bladder for the ultrasound test that will be done prior to the amniocentesis, so do not urinate before the test. You will lie on your back and some jelly-like material will be applied to your abdomen. A device will be passed over your abdomen. This device produces sound waves that you cannot hear. These sound waves will make an outline of your baby on the screen and will take a picture of the baby. This test will allow you to see your baby inside your uterus.

Interactive Activity: How do you teach material containing the danger signs of pregnancy without alarming the client? How do you know they learned? What kinds of written materials or audiovisuals might be helpful?

This activity is for the student's self-awareness.

Situation: A 24-year-old woman, gravida 1, TPAL 0000 at 40 weeks gestation, has come to the birth setting because she thinks she is in labor. She tells you that she felt the baby "drop" over the last two weeks and that she has been having contractions for the past two hours. She reports that she has not had any fluid leaking from her vagina and that she does not think her membranes have ruptured. She says, "My contractions are coming every 15 minutes and they last for about 30 seconds. They don't change when I lie down or walk about. I think I saw some bloody show, but I'm not sure. Do you think my labor has started?"

1. What signs of true labor does this woman have?

> She is having regular uterine contractions; they have continued for two hours; and they do not stop when she walks or changes positions. She is possibly having bloody show, but the nurse must still confirm that. Feeling the baby drop (lightening) is a premonitory sign of labor, not a sign of true labor.

2. How can the nurse determine whether or not this is true labor?

> The definitive way is for the nurse to check the woman's cervix for baseline data, wait an hour or two, and then re-check it. Cervical dilation would indicate true labor. For more confirmatory data, the nurse could observe for bloody show and observe the uterine contractions to see if they become stronger, longer, and closer together. The nurse could also ask the woman to describe her contractions—that is, whether she feels them in the back and lower abdomen, or above the navel.

3. How should the nurse answer the woman's question about whether or not she is in labor?

> Say something like, "You certainly have some signs of true labor. We will need to check your cervix and observe you for a while to see if it is dilating. Then we'll know for sure."

4. The nurse does an abdominal assessment of the woman's contractions and determines that they are moderate in strength. The woman's vital signs are within normal limits and the fetal heart rate is 136 bpm (measured for one full minute following a contraction). She also performs a digital examination of the client's cervix and finds that it is dilated to 2 cm and 50% effaced. She checks again in an hour and finds that the cervical dilation is between 2 and 3 cm and that the cervix is now about 80% effaced. The uterine contraction pattern remains the same, except that the contractions are now 45-50 seconds in duration. The nurse performs a Nitrazine paper test and confirms that the woman's membranes are intact. What stage and phase of labor do these findings indicate?

   First stage, latent phase

5. Vandevusse (1999) has described additional P's or essential forces of labor. A few have been listed in this table. Describe the effect they may have on labor and what the nurse could do to assist the woman/family.

Additional P's	Effect	Nursing Assessment/ Interventions
Preparations by Mother, eg. Prenatal class attendance	May have additional coping strategies such as breathing methods, birth plan, and expectations	Discuss expectations, teach coping strategies, and provide information pertaining to pregnancy and the birth process.
Professional providers, eg. Presence of the nurse in labor	Nursing support has been demonstrated as an important element in increasing confidence and satisfaction with labor	Provide 1:1 nursing support as much as possible, coach the partner on strategies that he/she might attempt
Procedures, eg. Requiring a woman to wear a hospital gown in labor	If appropriate, the woman could be encouraged to choose what she wants to wear, have information about procedures and protocols and be included in decision-making.	Assist the woman in decision-making as much as possible to increase her satisfaction with labor

---

Situation: A.F. is a 20-year-old woman, G2 P1, who is in active labor when she comes to the birthing unit. She says that she did not attend childbirth preparation classes during either pregnancy. She does not have insurance and says that she wants to use as little medication as possible in order to keep the cost as low as possible. She is becoming quite uncomfortable, at times moaning during her contractions. The unit does not have a Jacuzzi or tub for a water bath; however, there is a shower in each labor room.

---

1. Consider two strategies that could be suggested to A.F./partner to break the cycle between fear and tension and then between tension and pain.

   Strategies to break the cycle between fear and tension include: Information about labor and birth, progress in labor, what to expect and nursing presence. Strategies to break the cycle between tension and pain include: breathing techniques, hot/cold compresses, back massage and use of the shower.

2. A.F. chooses the shower for an hour, which her partner with your help/coaching uses to decrease her back pain (shower head pointed to her back) and in different positions (alternating between standing and sitting). You check her frequently and assess her fetal heart rate. A vaginal examination determines that she is now 7-8 cm. and beginning to feel some rectal pressure. What strategies would you include now to decrease fear? Decrease pain?

   Information about normal labor progress, encouragement of her and her partner's coping strategies and different positions.

Pain: Pharmacologic Analgesia Answer Key

Situation: J.T., G2 P1, is in active labor. Her cervix is dilated to 5 cm. She is experiencing a great deal of anxiety and pain and is unable to stay in control and breathe through her contractions. She does not want an epidural, so the primary care provider has prescribed Morphine by PCA pump.

1. What benefits are there to J.T. to have medication in this form?

   She controls the amount that is given, rapid onset (IV route) and ability to maintain a continuous infusion.

2. How soon can J.T. expect some relief from her pain?

   five-ten minutes after the PCA pump is started depending on the dosage and initial bolus

3. What observations are important for the nurse to make after giving the medications?

   Effectiveness of medication

   Ability to understand how to use the PCA pump

   Vital signs particularly respiratory rate

   Hourly check of amount of medication used

   The nurse should verify labor progress before administering a narcotic as opiates may lessen a mother's natural tendencies to push and can alter (slow) progression of birth.

4. Because of the side effects of these medications, what nursing diagnosis is needed in order to plan safety measures for J.T.?

   Risk for respiratory depression of infant at birth

5. What important nursing interventions are needed to address this nursing diagnosis?

   Have human and equipment resources available for neonatal resuscitation.

6. What contraindications are there to use of a PCA pump in labor?

   Allergy to medication and inability to speak English (family/partner cannot operate pump)

Situation: A 30-year-old woman is in active labor. She is a gravida 3, TPAL: 1011. Her cervix is dilated to 6 cm and is completely effaced. Her membranes are intact. She is complaining of pain with her uterine contractions (an eight on a scale of 0 to 10)and is asking for an epidural.

---

1. What are the advantages of having an epidural block (as compared with a systemic narcotic analgesic)?

   The woman will be alert and able to follow instructions. Good pain relief can be achieved, as a rule. Respiratory depression does not occur unless there is inadvertent systemic absorption of the medication. Gastric emptying is not delayed. Fetal distress is rare (but can, of course, occur).

2. What are the disadvantages of having an epidural block?

   The woman must have an IV line. Her legs will be at least partially immobile, so she will be confined to the bed. She may have difficulty emptying her bladder, and will need to void in a bedpan. There is some research that suggests that epidural analgesia may increase the incidence of longer labor and operative birth. Because a fairly large amount of medication is used in the epidural route, there is the risk of adverse reactions or rapid absorption of the anesthetic, resulting in maternal hypotension, convulsions, or paresthesia. Severe maternal hypotension also causes fetal distress.

3. Why is a spinal anaesthetic most often used for Caesarean births?

   Rapid onset, higher pain block and ability to provide epidural morphine for postpartum pain relief.

4. This client has a nursing diagnosis of pain related to processes of labor. What are appropriate outcomes for this diagnosis?

> **Client will express absence of pain with uterine contractions.**
>
> **Client will express satisfaction with her labor and birth experience.**
>
> **Client will remain relaxed and "in control" with uterine contractions.**

5. What important nursing interventions performed prior to the insertion of the epidural can prevent hypotension and fetal bradycardia?'

> **IV bolus and accurate baseline assessments of SP and P as well as FHR (q 5minutes X3 initially).**

Situation: A woman is in active labor at 41 weeks +5 days with an oxytocin induction. Her cervix is dilated to 4 cm and her membranes are intact. The FHR and uterine contractions are being monitored by an external electronic fetal monitor. The nurse notes a fetal heart rate of 110 beats per minute with adequate variability. There are no decelerations, but there are occasional accelerations up to a rate of 135/minute that last for 30 seconds.

1. Which data should be interpreted as positive signs?

   "Adequate" variability is positive; "good" variability would be better. Occasional accelerations are a positive sign. It is positive that there are no decelerations.

2. One hour later, the only change in the monitor strip is that the FHR variability has decreased and is now described as "minimal." The woman is describing contractions that are increasing in strength but due to her size (>250 lb), it is difficult to assess her contractions. An internal fetal scalp electrode would be beneficial in assessing her uterine activity. What must occur prior to its insertion?

   Rupture of the membranes

3. After the internal fetal scalp electrode is placed, you note that her contractions are frequent (>5 in 10 minutes) and now there are variable decelerations that occur with each contraction. What actions would be appropriate at this time?

   Discontinue oxytocin, turn to left side, administer oxygen and notify care provider.

Situation: : A woman has just been admitted to the assessment area (triage) of the birthing unit. The nurse has taken her vital signs and has completed a brief general systems review. The nurse now intends to perform Leopold's maneuvers as part of her assessment.

1. What information can the nurse obtain by doing Leopold's maneuvers?

    Fetal lie, position, presenting part and attitude. Best position for FHR assessment.

2. What should the nurse do before actually palpating the woman's abdomen?

    Explain the procedure.

    Wash her/his hands with warm water.

    Instruct the woman empty her bladder.

    Place the woman in supine position with a small pillow under her head. Her knees should be slightly flexed.

3. How many times should the nurse perform this procedure during the labor? Would all of the maneuvers be complete with each assessment?

    The nurse should perform the first and second maneuvers during labor. The first maneuver determines whether the fetal head, feet, or buttocks are in the fundus. The second maneuver determines the locates the back of the fetus.

4. What should the nurse do after completing the procedure?

Reposition the client for better placental blood blow. Auscultate fetal heart rate and examine fetal heart rate monitoring pattern during the procedure.

Document the findings obtained from the Leopold's assessment.

Auscultate the fetal heart rate (FHR).

Document the findings obtained from the examination.

5. The Leopold's assessment might likely be challenging to perform for which women?

The Leopold's maneuvers are most difficult to perform in women who are obese, in the first trimester of pregnancy, or who have polyhydramnios.

Situation: : Elise arrives at the birthing center after being in labor for six hours. Her cervix is dilated to 4 cm and she is having mild contractions, occurring every 5-10 minutes and lasting for 50-60 seconds. The external monitor shows a FHR of 130 bpm with moderate variability. When her membranes rupture, the fluid is heavily stained with meconium.

1. How would you describe rupture of membranes to her as a first sign of labor?

> **Some women will experience rupture of the fetal membranes as a first sign of labor. This occurs as either a sudden gush of amniotic fluid from the vagina or may occur as a slow leakage. In this case, it is common for the woman to be unsure whether the loss of fluid is amniotic fluid or urine. A sterile vaginal exam or test of vaginal secretions with nitrazine paper will indicate the presence of ammonitic fluid.**

Situation: Elise arrives at the birthing center after being in labor for six hours. Her cervix is dilated to 4 cm and she is having mild contractions, occurring every 5-10 minutes and lasting for 50-60 seconds. The external monitor shows a FHR of 130 bpm, with moderate variability. When her membranes rupture, the fluid is heavily stained with meconium.

2. How would the nurse explain the meconium-stained fluid to Elise/partner?

> **Amniotic fluid should be clear. If it is greenish in color, then the infant would have passed meconium stool in utero. This can indicate the unborn infant is stressed prior to birth, which could indicate fetal anoxia or other complications. The passage of meconium also occurs when the infant is postmature or positioned breech because of compression of the buttocks in the vaginal vault.**

3. What nursing assessments would the nurse include in her care when the membranes ruptured?

Documentation of time, color and amount of fluid, fetal heart rate, presence of contractions.

4. What initial preparations would the nurse include in her equipment for this baby's birth?

   Meconium aspirator and equipment for resuscitation/intubation, personnel trained for NRP.

5. Two hours later, her cervix is dilated only to 5 cm. Her contractions are still only mild-to-moderate and of the same frequency and duration. The decision is made to stimulate her labor with oxytocin (Pitocin). What would be the rationale for this decision?

   Concern regarding meconium-stained amniotic fluid and slow progress in labor.

Situation: : A 42-year-old woman in the 34th week of pregnancy is admitted to the birthing unit assesstion area because she is experiencing contractions. She is gravida 4, para 0; previous pregnancies have ended in miscarriage or preterm birth. Her cervix is dilated to 2-3 cm; uterine contractions are occurring every 5-10 minutes. She says, "I can feel the contractions, but they aren't painful." Electronic fetal monitoring, intravenous (IV) magnesium sulfate, and bed rest are ordered. Betamethasone (a glucocorticoid) is also ordered and is to be given intramuscularly (IM) immediately and repeated in 12 hours.

1. What risk factors does this woman have for preterm labor?

> **She is more than 40 years old (advanced maternal age).**
>
> **She has had previous preterm births.**

2. What assessments would the nurse in the assessment (triage) area of the birthing unit include in her care?

> **Abdominal assessment for presence of contractions, fetal heart rate (electronic fetal monitoring), documentation to ensure accuracy of her expected date of birth (EDB), and vital signs (SOGC<2000).**

3. What other symptoms of preterm labor are important for the nurse to assess? Why?

> The nurse should assess for other symptoms because they may:
> **(a) Indicate that the labor is progressing further**
>
> **(b) Provide data about client comfort needs. Symptoms include cramping, back pain, and pelvic pressure, and increased vaginal discharge or bloody show.**

4. What are contraindications or cautions for betamethasone therapy?

  - Chorioamnionitis is a contraindication for using betamethasone therapy.
  - Betamethasone is used with caution when tocolytics are needed.
  - Caution is indicated when the woman has maternal diabetes or multiple gestation (SOGC, 2000).

5. How should the nurse prioritize these interventions? (a) start the IV and begin administering the magnesium sulfate, (b) apply the external fetal monitor, (c) administer the betamethasone IM, (d) explain the need for bed rest and the other interventions. Explain your reasoning.

  - First, start the IV and begin the magnesium sulfate. The most important thing is to stop or slow the labor, if possible.
  - Next, administer the betamethasone. It requires a 24-hour period to become effective (and promote fetal lung maturity), and it is possible that this woman could give birth within 24 hours. At 32 weeks' gestation, this fetus is not likely to have mature lungs.
  - Next, apply the fetal monitor. It is important to have data about the fetal heart pattern and the uterine contractions, but no matter what the data indicates, the woman would still need the magnesium sulfate and the betamethasone. Monitoring can wait until those have been given.
  - Finally, do the necessary teaching, including the need for bed rest. Actually, the woman will need to be in bed in order to accomplish the preceding interventions anyway. After all the activity is over, the nurse can then reinforce the need to stay in bed and the rationale for it.

6. In general, how would this woman's care be different if she were at 22 weeks gestation?

  Emphasis would be on stopping the contractions. Betamethasone would not be given because a 20-week fetus is not viable. Fetal monitoring would be done to assure that the fetus is alive, not to determine fetal distress. For a fetus near term, fetal distress (non-reassuring fetal heart rate monitoring) might indicate the need for an emergency cesarean birth; there would be no point in that for a fetus prior to viability, particularly because surgical intervention poses an increased perinatal risk to the mother.

Situation: D.D. has come to the pre-admission clinic with her birth plan. She is gravida 1 TPAL: 0000. She has written on her plan that she does not want to have an episiotomy.

1. As the pre-admission nurse, how would you begin yor discussion with D.D. and her partner regarding episiotomy?

   Ask about their source of information regarding episiotomy; why it is important that she not have an episiotomy; and whether she has discussed it with her care provider

2. What would you suggest to D.D. that she could do antenatally to prevent an episiotomy?

   Investigate different positions for birth such as semi-sitting, side lying, squatting. Consider antenatal perineal massage. Practice breathing techniques from prepared childbirth class in preparation for working with the care provider during second stage.

Situation: D.D. is now in second stage labor. The fetus is quite large and the fetal monitor is showing early signs of fetal distress. As D.D. has already been in second stage labor for quite a while, it seems likely that she will need an episiotomy even though she has said that she would prefer not to have one.

3. What strategies might the nurse use to try and help D.D. achieve her goal of avoiding an episiotomy?

   Upright position, open-glottis pushing (pushing with woman's urges), warm compresses to the perineum and encouragement

4. If the physician or midwife determines that an episiotomy is required, what nursing measures will be needed postpartum?

> Education regarding the need for an episiotomy, application of ice to the perineum every 30 minutes, assessment of healing every shift, teaching regarding dissolving sutures and cleaning "front to back" with peribottle, sitz baths, etc.

Situation: T.J. is in labor. She is gravida 1 para 0. Her cervix is fully dilated, membranes are ruptured, contractions are strong, and T.J. has been pushing with them with little progress (descent). The fetus is engaged and in vertex position. The fetus is quite large and the fetal monitor is showing that the fetal heart rate is non-reassuring. The primary care provider has indicated that he/she has decided to do a forceps- assisted birth. When T. J. sees the forceps, she is afraid. She says, "Please be careful. You could crush my baby's head with those things!"

1. What nursing assessments should be made before the forceps are used?

    The nurse must assess the fetal heart rate (FHR) as a sign of fetal well-being.

    The nurse must be sure that the client's bladder is empty and catheterize her if necessary.

    It is also necessary for the presenting part to be engaged, the presentation to be vertex, the membranes to be ruptured, and that there be no CPD. However, the birth attendant usually makes these determinations.

2. Specifically, why must the nurse check, report, and record the FHR both before and after application of the forceps?

    The cord may be compressed between the fetal head and the forceps. A drop in the FHR would indicate that this had occurred, so the primary care provider would then remove and reapply the forceps. Forceps would be re-applied if the rate changed between the two.

3. What indicators are in place to facilitate the use of forceps?

    Engaged vertex position, membranes ruptured, cervix fully dilated

4. How will the health care provider likely describe the need for forceps in this situation?

    Prolonged second stage with slow descent of the presenting part, and non-reassuring fetal heart rate indicate that birth should occur quickly (SOGC, 2000).

Situation: M.J. is in second stage labor. She is gravida 1 para 0. Her cervix is fully dilated; the fetus is engaged and in vertex position. The fetus heart rate has decreased variability with variable decelerations. M.J. is very tired as she has been pushing for more than 1.5 hours. She is having trouble focusing and pushing with her contractions. The primary care provider tells M.J. and her partner that he/she will be using a vacuum extractor to assist with the baby's birth.

1. What conditions are present in this situation that have led to the decision to use the vacuum extractor to assist with birth?

   Maternal exhaustion, non-reassuring fetal heart rate, fetus in vertex position, and pushing in second stage without progress

2. List five contraindications for vacuum extration.

   Non-vertex presentations

   Incompletely dilated cervix

   Cephalo parietal disproportion (CPD)

   Mid-pelvic station

   Unengaged vertex presentation

3. Prior to the vacuum application, what two maternal assessments should the nurse make?

   Adequate pain relief and make sure that the bladder is empty

4. What documentation is critical?

   Time of application of the vacuum, time of birth, assessment of the newborn at birth including cephalohematoma, if present, and nursing care provided.

Situation: E. S. is in the 42nd week of gestation. Her fundal height is 38 cm. At 41 weeks, her fundal height was 39 cm, and at 40 weeks, it was 40 cm. Her primary care provider considers the pregnancy to be post-term and plans to induce labor. E. S. says, "I guess the baby will be even bigger than we expected. However, that's okay, since he's a boy. He can be a football player." The nurse replies, "Some post-term babies are larger than normal, but some are smaller. It is possible that your baby may not be especially large."

---

1. Which of the preceding data support the nurse's interpretation of E. S.'s situation?

   E. S.'s fundal height has been decreasing, which might mean that the fetus has stopped growing.

2. What else could E. S.'s decreasing fundal height indicate?

   Oligohydramnios-- deficiency in the amount of amniotic fluid

3. Based on ultrasound scanning, it is determined that E. S. does have oligohydramnios. However, an amnioinfusion is not planned. During labor what assessment will be crucial for the nurse to make?

   The nurse will need to pay close attention to the FHR pattern to determine whether variable decelerations occur. Oligohydramnios increases the risk of the umbilical cord being compressed by the fetal body, which would cause variable FHR decelerations. Other FHR patterns (e.g., loss of variability and late decelerations) may also occur, but variable decelerations are particularly associated with cord or head compression.

4. What special precautions should the nurse make for E. S.'s labor and birth?

   The nurse should be prepared for the need of a vacuum-assisted, forceps-assisted, or cesarean birth (and prepare E. S. for this mentally and emotionally, as well). The nurse

should also anticipate the need for neonatal resuscitation should the baby experience respiratory difficulty (e.g., as in meconium aspiration).

Situation: Ms. T., a G1 TPAL 0000, has been schduled for an induction using prostaglandin gel insertion at 41 weeks +5 days. She has had no signs of labour and is very anxious. She is to come to the birthing center at 0900 hours for the gel insertion but the unit is very busy. It is your responsibility, as the nurse in charge, to call her and inform her that you need her to postpone her arrival for approximately 6 hours until there is a bed and staff available to care for her. She is extremely upset and tells you that her partner has taken the day off work.

---

5. What would you include in your information to Ms. T. and her plan of care?

   Apology for the inconvenience caused by the unit business

   Questions regarding fetal movement counts (assessment of fetal health)

   Assessment of her understanding of prostaglandin gel insertion

   Questions regarding signs and symptoms of labor

Ms. T. comes in 6 hours later and prostaglandin gel is inserted as initially planned. Ms. T. has been monitored for 1 hour as per unit policy and there were no contractions noted or abdominally palpated and the electronic fetal monitor strip was reassuring. Mrs. T. is now able to go home over night and will return in the morning for reassessment and possibly an oxytocin induction.

---

6. What would you include in your teaching regarding warning signs and symptoms requiring return for assessment earlier than planned and information regarding an oxytocin induction?

   Warning signs and symptoms include: bleeding, contractions 5 minutes apart and becoming stronger, rupture of membranes and decreased fetal movement.

   Information about oxytocin should include: what it is (synthetic hormone), how it works, what the contractions may be like, options for pain relief and expectation regarding time of birth.

Situation: You are caring for a woman in labour and you have just assisted her to the bathroom. While on the toilet, she feels a "gush of fluid" and now "feels like something fell out".

1. Prioritize the following nursing interventions for this client. Explain your reasoning.

   _3_ Place the woman in Trendelenburg or knee-chest position.

   Place the bed in Trendelenburg or knee-chest position. (This could be #2, as discussed in the preceding step). It is essential to get pressure off the cord as quickly as possible.

   _4_ Use a gloved hand to push the fetal presenting part upward and keep it there until birth.

   Use a gloved hand and keep it there until birth. If this were done before #3, the nurse would have to remove her hand from the fetal part in order to change the bed position. Ideally, the nurse pushes the presenting part upward and maintains that position until the primary care provider orders it stopped (probably at delivery).

   _5_ Administer oxygen.

   Administer oxygen. It is important to increase maternal blood oxygen saturation to make more available to the fetus.

   _6_ Notify the primary care provider Stat.

   Notify the primary care provider Stat. The nurse probably will not call the primary care provider, but will rely on those who were summoned to help. However, the nurse should confirm that this has been done.

   _2_ Press or pull the call light for emergency assistance.

   A prolapsed is a true obstetric emergency. Activate the call light for emergency assistance. The nurse must continue to relieve compression of the cord by releasing pressure from the fetus against the umbilical cord. Restoring circulation to the infant is vital for neurologic outcome and survival.

   _1_ Inspect the perineum to see if the cord is visible.

   Inspect the perineum. It is necessary to confirm prolapse, or at least to have evidence it is suspected, before instituting the other measures.

 7 Assess the fetal heart rate.

> Assess the FHR. This should be done as soon as emergency measures have been taken. However, it should not precede them. If the FHR is being continuously electronically monitored, the nurse can glance at the monitor at any time during the other activities. The point is that the other activities must occur immediately, regardless of the information obtained from the fetal monitor.

Situation: A woman, gravida 3 para 2, at 20 weeks gestation, has been told that she is carrying twins. Her fundal height is greater than expected for the weeks of gestation. Although she states that she has experienced "quite a bit" of nausea and vomiting, she has gained 20 lbs already. The nurse auscultates a heart rate of 160 for Twin A and a heart rate of 140 for Twin B.

1. Evaluate the fetal heart rates.

   Both are within the normal limit of 110-160. It is normal for the rates to be different from each other.

2. The woman says, "Can you help me with my diet? I need to find a way to get everything the babies need, but still not take in so many calories. My friend only gained 25 lbs the whole time she was pregnant. I'm going to be too fat if I keep this up!" How should the nurse respond?

   The nurse should explain that (a) she will need more calories than would a woman carrying only one fetus, (b) that she can expect to gain more weight than her friend because she has two babies, not just one, and (c) ideally, she should plan to gain about 50 lbs during the pregnancy. She is about halfway through the pregnancy and still has about 30 lbs before the birth, even if she carries the baby 40 weeks. Remember, too, that many multifetal pregnancies are delivered prior to 40 weeks.

3. Which maternal vital sign is especially important to assess in this case? Why?

   Blood pressure. Multifetal pregnancy increases the risk of pregnancy-induced hypertension.

4. What should the nurse teach this woman about preventing preterm labor?

   The woman should avoid long periods of standing. She should cut back on the number of hours she works–certainly no more than 40 hours per week. She should schedule frequent rest periods during the day. She should ask family members or friends if they will care for her other children occasionally to allow her time to rest.

Situation: Ms. S., at G3 TPAL: 1011, comes in for a regularly scheduled office visit at 32 weeks gestation. She describes fatigue, increased slowness with intermittent backache, increased weight gain, decreased mobility and shortness of breath. She has her three-year-old with her. The fetal heart rates are 135/145 and you go on to assess her vital signs as well.

5. Place a mark beside each symptom describing whether it is normal for a multifetal pregnancy or abnormal and merits further assessment.

> **Fatigue: Normal**
>
> **Decreased mobility: Normal**
>
> **Weight gain of 30 lb. at 32 weeks: Normal**
>
> **Shortness of breath at rest: Abnormal. Although a multifetal pregnancy will cause pressure on the diaphragm and reduce the lung expansion of the pregnant woman, shortness of breath at rest is an indication of cardiovascular compromise and insufficiency of the heart to meet the circulation and oxygenation needs. This sign is an indication for a thorough physical evaluation.**
>
> **FHR 135/145: Normal**
>
> **Slight edema in her ankles: Normal**
>
> **BP 150/100: Abnormal. This finding indicates pregnancy-induced hypertension, which is not uncommon in the multifetal pregnancy. This pregnancy must be monitored closely and blood pressure reduced for fetal and maternal well-being.**

Ms. S. states that she is having trouble coping with this pregnancy and with her toddler and asks about community resources both for the last few weeks of pregnancy and for postpartum.

6. What would you tell her?

> **There are various prenatal support groups available in many communities, including Lamaze International (www.lamaze-childbirth.org), Maternity Center Association (www.maternity.org), International Childbirth Education Association (www.icea.org), and La Leche League International (www.lalecheleague.org).**

Situation: R. C., a primigravida, has been in prolonged, active labor. She is becoming exhausted. The primary care provider diagnoses cephalopelvic disproportion (CPD), and preparations are being made for a cesarean birth. R. C. and her partner are very worried about the need for surgery and are asking many questions. She says, "I've never been in a hospital before, much less had surgery." R. C. already has an IV, which was inserted early in her labor. The nurse inserts an indwelling urinary catheter. Waiting until the epidural/spinal is in place prior to inserting the urinary catheter is kinder to the woman.

1. What is the purpose of the indwelling catheter?

   Because of the location of the surgical incisions, it is important to keep the bladder empty to minimize surgical trauma.

   R. C. will not be able to get out of bed to go to the bathroom for several hours after surgery. Normal postpartum diuresis, as well as the large volume of IV fluids she will probably receive, will cause her bladder to fill rapidly.

2. The nurse makes a nursing diagnosis of "anxiety related to lack of knowledge about procedures and uncertain outcome for self and baby." What nursing interventions might be used to promote family-centered care and decrease anxiety? List at least 7.

   • **Explain all procedures as they are being performed.**

   • **Explain what to expect in the surgical suite.**

   • **Stay with the couple; do not leave them alone.**

   • **Help them to verbalize their anxiety (e.g., "This must be frightening for you," or "Tell me what you're thinking").**

   • **Provide realistic reassurance, when possible (e.g., if it is true, the nurse might say, "Your baby's heart rate looks good," or "I know you're very tired, but your pulse and blood pressure are still good").**

   • **Maintain a calm approach, as unhurried as the situation allows.**

   • **Control the environment: keep lights low, reduce noise, and limit unnecessary visitors and staff.**

3. The nurse positions R. C. in supine position on the operating table, with a small pillow under her head. She secures her legs and arms with safety straps, and applies a grounding pad. Evaluate the nurse's actions. What, if anything, needs to be changed?

The nurse should either tilt the operating table to one side or place a wedge under one of R. C.'s hips to keep the weight of the uterus off the vena cava and prevent hypotension. Begin preheating the radiant heater and notify the neonatal team per institutional protocols (varies).

4. After the birth, the nurse goes to visit the family. R.C. has many questions about what occurred prior to and during the surgery. How is this debriefing helpful for R.C. and her family?

As pain control may be a likely factor contributing to the client's discomfort, the nurse should inform the client to ask for pain medication when needed. Additionally, the client may have a patient-controlled analgesia (PCA) device, where she can deliver a safe dose of pain medication through her IV or epidurally as needed. Family should be encouraged to visit and provide support; however, they should also be educated about the client's need for frequent rest periods to coincide with the newborn's sleep/wake cycle. The client's discharge teaching related to her surgical procedure includes incisional care, family support, lifting restrictions to prevent complications to the incision, and information regarding follow-up care with her primary care provider.

Situation: A woman with borderline CPD is being given a trial of labor. The nurse is closely monitoring her cervical dilation and the uterine contractions.

1. Why is information about both cervical dilation and the uterine contractions essential to making judgments about CPD?

   Cervical dilation must occur in order for labor to progress. However, lack of dilation does not necessarily indicate CPD. Failure to dilate may, for example, be caused by ineffective or infrequent uterine contractions. If the contractions are strong, yet the cervix is not dilating, this is an indication of CPD.

2. What other regular observation must be made in order to determine whether the labor is progressing satisfactorily?

   The nurse must also perform a vaginal exam to assess fetal station (fetal descent). If the fetus does not descend in the presence of good contractions, vaginal birth will not occur.

3. After the woman is in sitting position for a period of time, the nurse helps her to assume a squatting position. The woman's membranes rupture; on vaginal exam, the woman's perineum is observed to be bulging and a small area of the fetal head is visualized. What does this mean?

   It indicates that the head has passed through the obstructed (contracted) area of the pelvis and that vaginal birth is likely.

Situation: Ms. S., a G1, TPAL: 0000, patient has been 3-4 cm. dilated, 100% effaced and -3 station with intact amniotic membranes for the last 2 hours. She is contracting every 5 minutes, coping well but is discouraged about her labour progress.

4. What risk factors does Ms. S. have for CPD?

   Lack of progress in labor, lack of descent in labor, and primigravida

5. What other information might assist with this diagnosis?

   Ultrasound reports, abdominal palpation, vaginal examination, antenatal records documenting prenatal care

6. What strategies might the RN suggest to facilitate progress in labor?

   Position change, walking, pain management, praise, information regarding a suggested time limit until re-assessment to decrease discouragement

Situation: P.K. is 20 years old. She is gravida 1 para 0, and at 41 weeks gestation. She is in active first-stage labor. Her cervix is dilated to 6 cm. Her uterine contractions are strong; frequency is every 5 minutes, duration is 70 seconds. The FHR is 120 with decreased variability and frequent variable decelerations. The decision is made to apply a fetal scalp electrode in order to better evaluate the FHR. When the amniotomy is performed, about 750 mL of green-tinged fluid with small white particles is obtained.

1. What information should the nurse include when charting this event?

    Time of amniotomy, FHR, and a description of the fluid

2. In preparation for this birth, the nurse should follow neonatal resuscitation principles. List 5 pieces of equipment that should be checked and ready for this baby's birth:

    Meconium aspirator

    Endotracheal tube 3.5 and 4.0

    Suction catheter

    Oxygen equipment

    Stethoscope

3. At the time of birth, the decisions regarding care are determined by the conditon of the baby and whether he/she is vigorous. What is included in this definition?

    Lusty cry, HR>100 and breathing

4. Describe the nursing care if the baby is vigorous at birth.

   Supportive care includes drying, warming, vital signs, and assessments as per protocol.

5. Describe the nursing care if the baby is not vigorous at birth.

   Begin the ABCs of resuscitation: establish airway, begin positive pressure ventilation, and cardiac compressions as needed.

Situation: C. L. is having labor augmented with oxytocin. Her cervix is 5 cm dilated and fully effaced and her membranes have ruptured. She is being continuously monitored for uterine activity and fetal heart rate.

1. What safety measures should the nurse take when setting up and administering the oxytocin? Explain the rationale for each.

   The oxytocin should be administered via a secondary (piggyback) line so that it can be turned off in an emergency without discontinuing the primary line, which may be needed to administer fluids and other medications.

   The oxytocin is diluted in 500 mL of fluid. Oxytocin must be given in very small doses (e.g., starting dosage is usually 0.5 to 2 mL/min) to prevent uterine hyperstimulation, so it must be greatly diluted.

   The oxytocin is administered by infusion pump so that there is no risk of overdosing the woman (as there would be with gravity/drip administration).

   The oxytocin is diluted in a physiologic electrolyte-containing fluid (not dextrose and water) because there is increased risk of water retention/intoxication when dextrose and water are used.

   The nurse labels the secondary bag and line with an orange or red "medication added" label in order to prevent accidental or unintended administration.

   The nurse places the woman in side-lying position to promote uterine blood flow.

   The nurse monitors the FHR and uterine contractions continually for signs of fetal distress or maternal complications, including uterine rupture, precipitous labor/delivery, cervical laceration, and uterine tetany.

2. The monitor shows that C. L.'s contractions are now every 3 minutes lasting 90 seconds with no relaxation of the uterus between contractions.. What should the nurse do first?

   Turn off the Pitocin. This eliminates the cause of the uterine hyperstimulation.

3. Match the letters of the information in the left column with the correct medication. Some letters may be used for more than one medication.

_C_ Laminaria	a. Stimulates contractions of uterine smooth muscle
_A, B, D_ Prostaglandin E gel/ suppository	b. Softens the cervix
_A, D, E_ Oxytocin (Pitocin)	c. Dilates the cervix mechanically
	d. Can cause uterine hyperstimulation
	e. Administered intravenously via infusion pump

Situation: A woman is to have her labor induced at 39 weeks gestation. However, a Bishop score indicates that her cervix is not "ripe." Therefore, she is to have prostaglandin gel inserted intravaginally prior to the induction. She asks the nurse, "Why are you putting that stuff in me? Do I have a vaginal infection?"

4. How should the nurse respond?

   The nurse should tell the woman the prostaglandin gel is not used to treat infection. This gel is intended to soften her cervix so that it will dilate more readily when the oxytocin is administered.

Case Study: The Client in First Stage Labor

Situation: A 30-year-old client, G1 P0, is in labor. Her cervix is dilated 4-5 cm and 75% effaced. Her membranes are currently intact. She has received routine prenatal care and her pregnancy has been uncomplicated.

Primary care provider's orders include:

- NPO with ice chips
- IV D5NS at 100 cc/hour
- Demerol 50 mg intramuscular for pain
- Continuous external fetal monitoring

Assessment findings reveal:

- Client is discouraged, tired, diaphoretic and restless.
- She is complaining of pain and is asking about options for pain relief medication.

Instructions: Prioritize **four** nursing interventions as you provide care for the client. Write the number in the box to indicate the order of your interventions (#1 = first, #2 = second, etc.) and briefly state your rationale for each intervention.

INTERVENTIONS	PRIORITY	RATIONALE
Promote relaxation.	3	Relaxation and comfort measures enhance the client's ability to cope with pain and reduce fear and anxiety.
Provide comfort measures, including pain relief, as ordered.	1	Pain increases fear. Fear increases anxiety. Anxiety and fear increase pain. Breaking the cycle enables the client to cope more easily.
Provide strategies for coping in 2nd stage labor.	4	Familiarity with what should be expected decreases fear-pain-anxiety.
Increase contact time with client.	2	Positive attitude and support from staff decreases anxiety.

About 45 minutes later, after pain medication has been administered, assessment data reveals:

- Contractions every 2-3 minutes lasting 60-90 seconds
- The client is complaining of nausea.
- States she, "Can't go on with this."
- Membranes ruptured

Interactive activity: With a partner, select the client concerns of highest priority and list the nursing interventions you would perform to meet client needs at this time

CLIENT CONCERNS	NURSING INTERVENTION
Anxiety related to progression of labor and fear of the unknown	1. Stay with client. 2. Increase positive reinforcement and reassurance. 3. Do less talking and explaining to client. 4. Assist client with energy self-preservation.

Situation: C.J. gave birth to her baby at 8 a.m. The nurse's assessment findings at 8 p.m. are as follows: B/P 120/80, pulse 70, respirations 16, temperature 99.5 o F, uterine fundus 1 cm above the umbilicus and right of midline, breasts are soft. C.J. says she has been perspiring a lot.

---

1. Which of the nurse's findings need to be explored further–that is, which findings could be an indication that a problem is developing?

   Temperature of 99.5° F

   Uterine fundus 1 cm above the umbilicus and right of midline

   C.J.'s report of lots of perspiration

2. What is probably causing C.J.'s slightly elevated temperature?

   Her temperature is not high enough to indicate infection, although that cannot be ruled out for certain. However, a slightly elevated temperature is normal in the early postpartum period. It may be a result of the increased metabolism from the work of labor and/or slight dehydration.

3. What other information does the nurse need in order to interpret the meaning of C.J.'s temperature reading?

   The nurse needs information about C.J.'s hydration status: her skin turgor and her intake and output. She also needs to assess for any signs of infection (e.g., urinary tract, episiotomy), including infections unrelated to childbearing (e.g., C.J. may have an upper respiratory infection).

4. What further data does the nurse need in order to adequately interpret the meaning of "fundus 1 cm above the umbilicus and right of midline"?

> C.J.'s fundus is a little higher in the abdomen than expected at this time, and the fundus is usually midline. This probably means that C.J.'s bladder is full, and it may also mean that her uterus is not contracting firmly enough to prevent bleeding. The nurse needs to ask C.J. how long it has been since she has voided and if she feels she has been emptying her bladder completely. The nurse should inspect C.J.'s vaginal pad to determine whether there is an excessive amount of lochia. The case study does not provide information as to whether the uterus is boggy or firm to palpation; this, too, is needed in order to assess the implications of her fundal height and location.

5. The nurse is caring for a client in the immediate postpartum period. While assessing for each of these potential complications after delivery, which clinical manifestations will the nurse most likely identify? Match the clinical findings with the complication.

A, D — Postpartum hemorrhage	a. Uterus boggy and high in abdomen
A, B, C, G — Puerperal infection	b. Foul-smelling lochia
E, H — Urinary tract infection	c. Temperature of 102° F
F, I — Thrombophlebitis	d. Large amount of lochia rubra, blood in the bed
	e. Burning with urination
	f. Quarter-sized red, warm area on calf
	g. Abdominal and pelvic pain
	h. Frequent urination
	i. Pain with dorsiflexion

> *Urinary tract infection could also involve fever (typically low-grade) and pain (usually flank pain), but frequent and burning urination are the classic signs/symptoms.

Situation: A woman has just given birth to her first baby. She wishes to breastfeed her baby, but she has not been to any parent education classes. She says, "I don't even know how to begin."

1. Write a nursing diagnosis for this woman.

   Risk for ineffective breastfeeding related to lack of knowledge of breastfeeding techniques

2. Write goals/expected outcomes for this nursing diagnosis.

   The infant will latch on, suck, and swallow properly (nutritive sucking).

   The infant will average 15 minutes total per feeding, with nutritive sucking.

   The mother will demonstrate breastfeeding techniques that have been taught (e.g., to remove the infant from the breast if infant is "chewing" instead of sucking and swallowing).

   The mother will verbalize satisfaction with breastfeeding.

   The mother will verbalize confidence in her ability to breastfeed.

3. The woman asks, "How long should I let the baby nurse on each breast?" What should the nurse tell her?

   It may take five minutes for the milk-ejection (let-down) reflex to occur at first. If the baby is positioned and sucking correctly, there is no need to limit time at the breast. Improper positioning rather than length of time at the breast usually causes nipple trauma. If the woman insists on a general guideline for time at the breast, the nurse can tell her to start with about 10 minutes on each side, changing sides when the infant ceases to nurse vigorously. It is important to have the infant nurse long enough to empty the first breast, yet avoiding prolonged "snacking" and non-nutritive nursing.

4. What should the nurse teach the woman about techniques preventing nipple trauma?

Properly position the baby for nursing.

Avoid plastic bra liners that keep the nipples moist.

Use disposable bra pads to absorb leaking milk; change them frequently so that they are not wet.

Do not use soap on the nipples.

Use a variety of positions for feeding.

Insert a finger between the baby's mouth and the breast to break the suction before removing the baby from the breast.

Leave the flaps of her nursing bra down for a few minutes after feedings.

5. On the first postpartum day, the woman says, "I've heard that my milk won't come in for two or three days. Is there any point in letting the baby breastfeed now? Will the baby even get anything?" What should the nurse tell her?

It is important for the baby to nurse because this stimulates milk production. The client is correct that the breasts will not produce milk for two or three days; however, they do produce colostrum, which contains antibodies, protein, and fat-soluble vitamins that nourish the baby until the milk comes in.

Situation: Ms. R., a recent immigrant from India, has given birth to her first child. She wishes to breastfeed but states that her mother has advised her that colostrums is harmful to the baby. She wishes to begin breastfeeding when her "milk comes in" around the third day.

6. What information does Ms. R. need in order to make an informed choice regarding infant nutrition?

Information on supply and demand, benefits of colostrum and breastfeeding

7. What options might you explore with her?

   Pumping to increase her milk supply, an interpreter to ensure that she understands your information, referring her to public health for follow-up in the community

8. What follow-up would be important to her decision to breastfeed?

   Community support

Situation: A 16-year-old gave birth to a baby boy three hours ago. It was a vaginal birth and she has a midline episiotomy and hemorrhoids. She asks the nurse to take her baby to the nursery for a few hours, saying, "Please take care of it for a while. I am exhausted. I was in labor for 16 hours and had no sleep at all last night. I really need to sleep." The baby is lying across the mother's lap and the mother does not enfold the baby before handing him to the nurse.

1. What signs (defining characteristics) of delayed bonding is the mother of exhibiting?

   She is not holding the baby close. She is calling him "it" instead of "him" and is not using his name.

2. What risk factors are present that should alert the nurse to the possibility of delayed bonding?

   She is a teenager; she is fatigued and in pain.

3. Is there enough data to infer that there is an attachment/bonding problem?

   No. The mother may just be tired.

4. What would be an appropriate nursing diagnosis for this situation?

   Risk for Altered Parent/Infant Attachment related to developmental level, fatigue, and pain

5. Prioritize the mother's needs at this time. Explain your thinking.

      1   Sleep and rest

      2   Interaction time with the baby to facilitate bonding

      3   To learn how to hold and cuddle the baby

First, sleep and rest; the other two can be done after she is rested.

This mother is exhibiting some signs of delayed bonding, and her age may mean that she needs additional support in making adaptations to parenthood. However, she cannot be expected to progress with emotional adaptations until her physical needs (e.g., sleep and rest) are met. Until she is rested, the nurse cannot adequately assess the bonding.

6 What are the important nursing interventions for this woman at this time? Explain your thinking.

Role model how to cuddle the baby and call him by name.

Take the baby to the nursery.

Explain that it is important to spend time with the baby during the first 24 hours after birth.

Assess for other signs of delayed bonding.

Rationale: The most important activity at this time is to take the baby to the nursery so the mother can sleep. The nurse should also cuddle the baby and call him by name as she takes him from the mother; however, this is less important than her need for rest at this time. The woman is not receptive to explanations at this time and cannot bond well when she is exhausted. Assessment of the bonding should continue throughout the woman's stay in the birthing unit.

7. After the mother is rested, what other physical condition will the nurse need to assess for to be sure that it is not interfering with the mother's ability to bond?

Episiotomy pain

Situation: A 16-year-old gave birth to a male infant 6 hours ago. You are the nurse providing care to this new mother and her infant. The mother and infant's vital signs are stable. You bring the portable bathtub to the bedside for the baby's first bath after discussion with the teenage mother. She is tired but eager to learn how to care for her infant.

Describe eight things that could be incorporated in this interactive bathing opportunity.

1. Call the infant by name.

2. Encourage the mother's efforts in care by helping and giving suggestions rather than doing the bath.

3. Praise her efforts in bathing.

4. Model behavior, such as cuddling and holding.

5. Describe the newborn's abilities such as vision, hearing, and touch.

6. Describe important features of the bath such as drying the cord after the bath.

7. Treat her with respect during the bath.

8. Describe the newborn preference for voice and range of sound preferred.

Postpartum Hemorrhage and Disseminated Intravascular Coagulation (DIC) Answer Key

Situation: N.C., a 35-year-old multipara gave birth to a 9 lb. 14 oz. baby two hours ago after a rapid labor. She has saturated three peripads since the birth. Her fundus is firm and at the level of the umbilicus. Her vital signs are within normal limits.

1. Which data should alert the nurse that N.C. is at risk for postpartum hemorrhage?

   Large infant, rapid labor, multiparity

2. The risk factors for postpartum hemorrhage have been described as the 4 Ts. What are they?

   T-thrombus (abnormalities of coagulation, e.g. hemophilia, DIC)

   T-tone (over-distended uterus, e.g. multiple gestation) (uterine muscle exhaustion, e.g. rapid labor)

   T-tissue (retained products or placental fragments)

   T-trauma (precipitous delivery, lacerations of the cervix or vagina)

3. At the next assessment, the nurse determines that N.C.'s fundus is soft. Other data are unchanged. What are the priority interventions? Explain your reasoning.

   Be sure that N.C. does not need to void because a full bladder can cause uterine atony.

   If the bladder is not distended, massage the uterus and attempt to express any clots. This may stimulate the uterus to contract to compress blood vessels at the placental site and stop excessive bleeding. The nurse should continue to assess the fundus, lochia, and vital signs frequently. If the uterus does not become firm on massage, the nurse should notify the care provider.

4. After the nurse performs the interventions in #3, N.C. continues to bleed heavily. The nurse notifies the primary care provider, administers 20 units of oxytocin through her IV line according to protocols, and continues to monitor the bleeding. What are the most important vital signs to monitor at this time? Why?

> **Pulse and blood pressure**
>
> **The woman is at risk for hypovolemic shock because of the bleeding.**

5. The nurse also implements a medical order to insert an indwelling urinary catheter. What is the rationale for doing this?

> **Because of the blood loss and risk for hypovolemic shock, it is essential to evaluate the woman's tissue perfusion. Urine output is a good indicator of kidney perfusion and fluid balance. In addition, the woman will probably be too weak to get out of bed to go to the bathroom.**

Case Study: The Client Diagnosed with Postpartum Hemorrhage

Situation: Six hours ago, a 29-year-old client (gravida 3, para 3) vaginally gave birth to a male infant. About two hours after delivery, the client began to bleed steadily and the estimated blood loss currently is about 700 mL. Thus far, the client has received one unit of blood and presently is receiving IV fluids at 150 cc per hour. She has a Foley catheter in place. Vital signs at 2 pm are: BP 100/60, P 100, and R 12. Hematocrit is 24%. You are assigned to care for the client on the postpartum unit during the evening shift.

Instructions: Prioritize the nursing interventions you would perform when providing care for the client. Write the number in the box to identify the order of your interventions (#1 = first, #2 = second, etc.)

INTERVENTIONS	PRIORITY #
Assess uterus for consistency, firmness, and position.	2
Monitor urine output. Assess accurately intake and output.	5
Note amount and character of lochia.	3
Assess breath sounds.	4
Take vital signs.	6
Review lab values.	7
Explain plan of care to woman/family	1

The client has laboratory work done on your shift and a repeat hematocrit at eight hours post-delivery is 29%. She receives another unit of blood.

Instructions: Based on the lab data, identify the priority problem and the nursing interventions for this situation.

PROBLEM

1. Potential hypovolemic shock
2. Related to blood loss

NURSING INTERVENTIONS

- Maintain open IV.
- Measure intake and output.
- Assess skin for pallor, perfusion, and coldness.
- Take vital signs and monitor lochia and fundal tone.
- Obtain appropriate labs.

Which information would indicate that the client's condition is improving?

- BP and vital signs stable
- Hemoglobin and hematocrit rising
- Small amount of lochia without clots
- Uterus firm
- Indwelling urinary catheter removed
- Intravenous removed

Three days after birth the client's hematocrit is 33% and she is not experiencing any abnormal bleeding. She is planning to be discharged the next day.

Instructions: Work with a partner to develop a discharge-teaching plan for the client.

- Expect the return of bright red or dark red blood after the 4th postpartum day.
- Report fever over 100.4° F.
- Report foul-smelling lochia.
- Report painful urination.
- Remind the client that she'll need to rest and attend to diet to rebuild her iron store.
- Eat foods that are high in iron.

Situation: An obese woman is admitted to the postpartum unit after a cesarean birth. The cesarean was performed for fetal distress after a 16-hour labor. Her history includes two prior miscarriages and prolonged rupture of membranes before this birth. Two days after the birth, the nurse observes that the edges of her abdominal incision are not approximated; the skin around the incision is red and the wound is draining a small amount of seropurulent drainage. The wound is painful and tender to touch.

1. What risk factors for infection are present?

   Obesity

   Long labor

   Cesarean birth

   Prolonged rupture of membranes

2. What symptoms of infection are present?

   Abdominal incision is not approximated

   Skin around the incision is red

   Seropurulent wound drainage

3. What other assessments should the nurse make that are related to puerperal infection?

   The nurse would want to know if the infection is a localized wound infection or if other areas of the reproductive tract or abdomen are involved. The nurse should take the woman's temperature, assess uterine involution, assess the lochia for odor, and inquire about flu-like symptoms such as fatigue and nausea.

4. What interventions will be initiated by the nurse?

Pain management, wound care, and more frequent assessments of temperature and wound

5. What other orders would be appropriate for this patient?

A culture of the drainage

Removal of some sutures to allow for drainage

Packing (e.g., iodoform gauze) may be placed in the wound

Broad-spectrum antibiotics may be given until a report of the culture returns

Warm compresses to the wound

Analgesics

Situation: Two weeks after giving birth, a woman calls the care provider's office because, she says, "Something is wrong with my breast." Upon further questioning, she says that she has a hot, hard, sore spot "about the size of a golfball" on her left breast. She says that she has been having chills and a headache.

1. What advice will be given to this woman?

   Come in for assessment and intervention as well as breastfeeding support.

2. What symptoms would lead the nurse to suspect mastitis instead of breast engorgement?

   Breast engorgement usually occurs earlier, and it usually involves both breasts. An engorged breast is usually hard, tender, and shiny over the entire breast, not just in one spot. A woman with breast engorgement usually does not feel ill or have chills and headache.

3. The woman says, "I think I may have an infection, so I've been bottle-feeding my baby so she won't get sick." What should the nurse tell her?

   Tell her to continue breastfeeding. It will not harm the baby, and weaning during engorgement may cause engorgement and stasis, leading to abscess formation.

4. What other advice should the nurse provide regarding follow-up, infant nutrition, and self care?

   The woman should see her primary care provider for definitive diagnosis and probable antibiotic therapy as soon as possible. Meanwhile, she should drink at least 3000 mL of fluids per day; continue breastfeeding or pumping her breasts, and use warm compresses or a warm shower to promote comfort.

Situation: Two postpartum clients have venous thrombosis. Client A has a history of varicose veins; her left leg has two warm, tender, red areas along the medial calf of her leg. The vein in that area is enlarged and hard, and the client says it hurts when she walks. Client B has pain in her left leg when she ambulates, and she says her leg "feels stiff." Her calf is swollen and her foot is edematous. Her leg is pale and cool to the touch, and the pedal and posterior tibial pulses are diminished.

1. Which client has superficial venous thrombosis?

   Client A

2. How is the care of these two clients similar?

   Both will be on bed rest initially.

   The leg may be elevated for both.

   Both will probably receive analgesics.

   Both may require elastic support hose after symptoms subside.

3. Which client is at most risk for a pulmonary embolus?

   Client B

4. What nursing interventions will Client B need that are not needed by Client A? Why?

   • **Monitor for signs of bleeding (because of anticoagulant therapy).**

- Advise the client to avoid aspirin and nonsteroidal anti-inflammatory drugs (because of anticoagulant therapy).

- Teach the client about the need for prolonged warfarin therapy on discharge from the hospital.

- On discharge, advise client to avoid long periods of standing and to wear support hose to prevent venous stasis.

- Client B has deep venous thrombosis, which requires long-term anticoagulant therapy. Deep venous thrombus is also more likely to recur and/or become chronic, so preventive measures are more important.

5. How would Client B's treatment be different if she were pregnant? Why?

She would not be given warfarin for long-term management of the thrombosis because it is teratogenic. She would, instead, be given subcutaneous heparin.

Situation: C.C. gave birth to a healthy, full-term baby girl after a somewhat difficult pregnancy. She was not married when she became pregnant, and at 10 weeks' gestation, she considered having an abortion. Her parents urged her to continue the pregnancy and marry the baby's father, which she did. However, even at her last prenatal visit, she was still anxious about the limitations that a baby would impose on her. Shortly before the birth, her husband was imprisoned for stealing a car. C.C. is unemployed and living on public aid; her parents do not have room in their trailer for her and the baby.

Five days after the birth of her baby, a home health nurse is visiting C.C. Her hair has not been combed and her body odor suggests that she has not been bathing. The nurse sees that the house is messy and dirty. When asked how she is doing, C.C. starts crying. She says, "I'm just so tired; and there's no one to help me. I am so mad at my parents for talking me into this!"

1. What data in C.C.'s history should alert the nurse that she is at risk for postpartum depression?

   Ambivalence and anxiety throughout the pregnancy

   Lack of social support and confidants

   Low income level

2. What symptoms of postpartum blues is C.C. exhibiting at this time? Which symptoms should be explored as possible symptoms of postpartum depression?

   Symptoms of postpartum blues: Crying, fatigue, anger (at her parents)

   The following symptoms may indicate more severe depression: C.C. is not attending to her personal hygiene or care of her environment. She verbalizes feelings of anger, exhaustion, and lack of support.

3. What other information does the nurse need in order to determine whether C.C.'s symptoms are normal or whether she may have postpartum depression?

> The nurse should try to determine if C.C.'s lack of hygiene and poor housekeeping are new symptoms, or if this is how she functioned before becoming pregnant. The nurse should assess the maternal-infant bonding. She should assess whether and how well C.C. is attending to the baby's needs (e.g., Is the baby clean? Is the baby being fed regularly?) She should ask C.C. more about her feelings (e.g., guilt, sadness) and her feelings about the baby. The nurse should ask C.C. whether her appetite has changed, and what she is eating. She should ask her if she cries often.

4. How can the nurse help C.C. at this time?

- The nurse could attend to the baby while C.C. takes a bath and attends to her personal hygiene.

- The nurse could either clean up the house or arrange for someone to come do it (if such help is available in the community).

- The nurse could contact any community agency that might provide help for C.C., either for childcare (e.g., Mother's Morning Out) or for emotional support.

- The nurse should tell C.C. to call her primary caregiver if any of the signs of postpartum depression develop (and leave her a written list of signs and symptoms).

- The nurse should find out whether C.C. has any friends who could at least serve as confidants, and advise her to call them.

- The nurse should determine whether C.C.'s parents are able and willing to provide support for her (e.g., housework, shopping, emotional support).

1. Match the descriptions to the correct newborn reflex.

a. When the nurse strokes the infant's palate, he begins to suck.	c. Babinski
b. When the nurse strokes the infant's cheek, the infant turns her head to that side.	f. Grasp
c. The infant's toes flare outward and the big toe dorsiflexes when the nurse strokes the lateral sole of its foot.	d. Moro
d. When the nurse raises the infant and then allows the head and trunk to drop back 30 degrees, the infant's arms and legs extend and abduct, the fingers fan open with the thumbs and forefingers forming a "C"; the arms then return to their normally flexed state.	b. Rooting
e. When the nurse claps her hands near the infant, the infant abducts the arms and flexes the elbows, similar to a Moro reflex	e. Startle
f. When the nurse touches the baby's palm near the base of the fingers, the hand closes into a tight fist.	g. Step
g. When the nurse holds the infant upright with the feet touching the bed, the infant lifts one foot and then the other.	a. Sucking
h. When lying on the back with head turned to one side, the infant extends the arm and leg on the same side and flexes the opposite arm.	h. Tonic neck

2. Which of the following newborns is not breathing normally? (There may be more than one.)

Baby A is breathing deeply, with a regular rhythm, at a rate of 40/min. This is normal.

Baby B is sleeping. He is breathing shallowly, at a rate of 26/min, with short periods of apnea. The normal respiratory rate for term infants at rest might be as low as 30. When the rate of breathing is slow, the infant should be assessed further for signs of respiratory distress or compromised oxygenation. Immediately after birth, mild irregularity in the pattern of breath will occur. This means brief periods of apnea less than 10 seconds in duration are considered normal. However, the nurse/parent needs to assess the infant closely for signs of true infant apnea or signs of respiratory distress.

Baby C is sleeping. He is breathing diaphragmatically and his sternum is retracting. The rate is 70/min. This infant is exhibiting signs of respiratory distress. While asleep the breathing rate should be approximately 30-50 breaths/min. Tachypnea is 70 breaths/min. Use of accessory muscles, such as diaphragmatic breathing or retractions, indicates the infant is experiencing dyspnea. This infant should be evaluated immediately and offered respiratory support.

Baby D is crying. He is breathing abdominally, irregularly, and at a rate of 70/min. This is normal for the crying baby. Although the respiratory rate is transiently high, it should return to normal (30-50) after the infant is calm. If the infant remains tachypneic, the nurse needs to conduct further respiratory assessment.

Baby E is breathing shallowly, with 40-second periods of apnea and cyanosis. Although the rate of breathing is normal, these findings indicate the infant is experiencing compromise to the oxygenation status. The infant showing signs of respiratory distress requires immediate intervention.

3. Why does the nurse need to count a newborn's apical pulse and respirations for a full minute?

Because they are irregular, counting for 30 seconds and multiplying by two (for example) would not be accurate.

Situation: A newborn (4 hours old) weighs 8 lb. and is 20 inches long. Her head is 12 inches in circumference and her chest is 14 inches in circumference. Her anterior fontanel is palpable; the posterior fontanel is not. Bowel sounds are present and she has just passed meconium. She has fine hair on her forehead and shoulders and vernix in the folds of her wrists, elbows, and ankles.

4. Why is it significant that the infant has passed meconium?

It indicates that the anus is patent with no obstruction of the bowel. The passage of stool is also a sign of normal peristalsis.

5. Which of the assessment findings may be cause for concern?

The baby's head is significantly smaller than her chest; the head should be slightly larger than the chest. Other findings are normal. The anthropometric measurements should be plotted on the newborn growth chart. Abnormal findings either above the 90% or below the 10%, should be remeasured. If reading is accurate, it is important to report the findings to the primary care provider.

1. A baby boy was born at 12:15 p.m. At 12:16 p.m., the nurse obtains an Apgar score of 8. When should the next Apgar assessment be performed?

   At 12:20 p.m. Apgars are performed at 1 and 5 minutes after birth. If the score is less than 8, a 10-minute assessment is performed and a score assigned.

2. One minute after birth an infant's heart rate is 60/min. The baby has slow respirations and a weak cry, slight flexion of extremities, grimaces when suctioned, and is pink except for the hands and feet, which are blue. What is the Apgar score?

   Answer: 5

   Heart rate =1

   Respiratory rate =1

   Muscle tone =1

   Reflex irritability =1

   Color =1

3. What nursing intervention is required for the infant in the preceding question?

   Gently stimulate the infant by rubbing his/her back; administer oxygen.

4. When assessed at five minutes after birth, the infant's heart rate is 110/min. The baby now has a strong cry, but still has minimal flexion of the extremities. The baby moves promptly when slapped gently on the sole of the foot. Color is unchanged: pink except for acrocyanosis. What is the 5-minute Apgar score?

> **Answer: 8**
>
> **Heart rate =2**
>
> **Respiratory rate =2**
>
> **Muscle tone =1**
>
> **Reflex irritability =2**
>
> **Color =1**

5. What nursing intervention is now required?

> **Nothing except continued observation and support of the infant's spontaneous efforts**

Situation: A baby girl has just been born. She is full term and weighs 7 lb. 8 oz. Her Apgar score is 8 at one minute.

1. Prioritize the following nursing activities in the immediate care of the baby.

   a. Place the infant skin-to-skin with the mother, in a warmer, or use any other method to prevent heat loss.

   b. Support respiratory adaptation: suction the mouth and then the nose.

   c. Perform a complete physical examination.

   d. Bathe the infant.

   e. Administer Ilotycin eye ointment.

   f. Assess the baby's respirations and heart rate.

   g. Footprint the baby and thumbprint the mother; apply matching identification bracelets.

   (b) The most urgent need is to support the infant's respiratory efforts.

   (a) The nurse can provide warmth and then assess the respirations and heart rate while the baby is in the warmer or on the mother's chest.

   (f) After supporting the respiratory efforts and ensuring warmth, the nurse can auscultate the heart and lungs to determine if more support is needed.

   (g) Identification measures should be attended to as soon as physiologic needs are met, but certainly within a few minutes after the birth. It must be done before mother or infant leave the birth area (e.g., to be transferred to a postpartum unit).

   (e) Administration of the eye ointment could be done next, or it could be postponed for a while to facilitate bonding.

   (c&d) The complete physical examination can be performed concurrently with the bath.

2. Write nursing interventions to help achieve the following goals for the infant:

    a. Respiratory adaptation:

        Place in Trendelenburg position.

        Suction nose and mouth.

        Assess respirations, heart rate, color, muscle tone, and irritability.

        Assess gestational age.

    b. Safety, including prevention of infection:

        Take rectal temperature.

        Administer eye ointment (e.g., Ilotycin).

        Administer aquamephyton (vitamin K).

        Place matching bracelets on infant and mother.

        Footprint infant; fingerprint mother.

    c. Thermoregulation:

        Dry well.

        Place hat on head.

        Place skin-to-skin with mother.

        Wrap warmly or place under warmer.

        Do not bathe infant until temperature stabilizes.

3. The parents ask you to explain the purpose of the eye ointment and Vitamin K. How would you describe the reason for their administration?

    Vitamin K is administered to newborns because their own bodies cannot produce it. This reduces the likelihood of bleeding disorders and stimulates their liver to produce the necessary clotting factors: II, VII, IX and X. Also, state laws currently require every infant receive erythromycin eye ointment prophylactically to prevent gonorrheal and chlamydial conjunctivitis. As the medication will likely cause mild irritation and blurring of vision to the newborn, the nurse may delay application for up to an hour after birth so the parents can bond with the infant.

1. Match the nursing interventions to the mechanism of heat loss they are meant to prevent.

Conduction d,e,h, i	a. Regulate room temperature to keep it in the thermal neutral zone.
Convection a,b,g	b. Keep a hat on the newborn's head.
Evaporation c,f	c. Dry the infant well after birth.
Radiation a,b,g	d. Warm hands and stethoscope before touching baby.
	e. Do not place crib close to a window or fan.
	f. Dry the baby well when bathing.
	g. Keep the infant well wrapped.
	h. Use a warm blanket to wrap the infant.
	i. Place infant skin-to-skin with mother when feeding.

Situation: A baby was born one hour ago after a precipitous birth. He weighed 7 lb. 8 oz. The baby's heart rate is 120 and respirations are 38. Auxiliary temperature, taken just after birth, was 98° F. The mother is holding the loosely wrapped baby, counting fingers and toes, and so on. The baby is lying with flexed arms and legs, and is not shivering. The mother points out to the nurse that the baby's hands and feet are blue.

2. What should the nurse do? Why?

> **Feel the hands and feet to see if they are cool. A bluish discoloration of the extremities (acrocyanosis) is normal at first, but if the extremities feel cool, the baby's temperature may be falling and the nurse will need to take the temperature. Explain all of this to the mother. Place newborn skin-to-skin with mother, cover the newborn with warm blankets and retake temperature in 30 minutes.**

3. What risk factors for hypothermia are present in the environment?

> **The only risk factor in the situation is that the infant experienced a precipitous birth.**

Situation: An average newborn infant weighs 8 lbs (3.64 kg).

---

1. How many calories per day does this baby need?

   Approximately 364-437 calories per day

   Newborns need 100-120 calories per kilogram per day. Multiply 3.64 by 100 to obtain an answer of 364 calories per day. Multiply 3.64 by 120 to obtain an answer of 437 calories per day.

2. If formula contains 20 kcal/ounce, how many ounces of formula will the newborn need per day?

   18-22 ounces. Divide 364 by 20 to obtain 18.2. Divide 437 by 20 to obtain 21.9.

3. If the newborn takes exactly 2 ounces at each feeding, how many feedings will be needed in order to take in 18-22 ounces (or the necessary number of calories)? Over a 24-hour period, how often would the baby need to eat?

   Nine to eleven feedings

   This would mean that the baby eats every 2-3 hours.

4. A new mother asks you to describe how much breast milk her baby is getting at a feeding and if it is enough for this infant. She explains that her mother who did not breastfeed is worried. How will you answer? How would your answer be different on Day 3 or at 2 weeks of age?

   Describe your answer in terms of feedings, calories, and output.

Situation: The parents of a newborn male infant have been asked if they wish to have their baby circumcised. They seem anxious and tell the nurse, "We don't really know if we should do this. We are afraid it will hurt him. Does he need to have it done?"

1. What nursing diagnosis is most appropriate?

   Anxiety related to uncertainty about effects of and need for the procedure. Alternatively, you might choose Decisional Conflict; however, that diagnosis focuses more on personal life values. In this case, once the parents have adequate information and are reassured about the procedure's relative safety, they will probably not have so much difficulty making their decision.

2. How can the nurse help decrease the parents' anxiety?

   Allow them to express their concerns.

   Share information about the risks and benefits of the procedure.

   Explain what, if anything, would be done to decrease the baby's pain during the procedure.

   Explain that the nurse will be there to comfort the baby during the procedure (if it is the chosen method).

3. The parents decide to have the baby circumcised. One hour after the procedure, they call the nurse to their room to show her a 1 x 2 cm spot of blood on the dressing covering the site. What should the nurse do?

   Assure them that this is normal, but that they are right to watch it. Ask them to call if the spot begins to bleed more.

4. Three hours after the circumcision, the parents again call the nurse. This time there is a 2 x 2 inch spot of blood on the dressing. What should the nurse do?

Apply intermittent gentle pressure to the site, using sterile gauze. Call the primary care provider.

5. The baby is dismissed to home care after 24 hours. The next day, the parents telephone the primary care provider's office to report that the baby's penis has "some yellow stuff" on it. They say that it is not bleeding and that they have been keeping petroleum jelly on the site, as instructed. When asked, they say that the yellow exudate does not have any odor. They ask, "What should we do? Try to wash it off? Bring him to see the doctor? What?" What should the nurse tell them?

Assure them that they were right to call and check, just to be safe. Tell them that this yellow exudate is normal on the second day. Also review the symptoms of infection and stenosis and tell them that they should feel free to call back if there is any question about how the penis is healing.

Situation: Twenty-four hours after delivery, and just prior to discharge, a male infant is about to undergo an elective circumcision. He has not been fed for several hours, and is restrained on a circumcision board. The procedure will be done using a Gomco clamp. The nursery nurse will provide care for the infant after the circumcision and prior to discharge.

Instructions: Identify the priority nursing interventions that should be included in the infant's post-circumcision care.

- **Monitor for first void because tissue edema may interfere with voiding.**
- **Dress circumcision wound with Vaseline gauze. This helps prevent the diaper from sticking to the penis.**
- **Check the circumcision site for bleeding. Scant amounts on the diaper are normal.**

With a partner, list the discharge instructions that should be given to the mother when providing circumcision care at home and give the rationale for the action.

INSTRUCTIONS	RATIONALE
Demonstrate application of petroleum jelly to the circumcision site.	This prevents irritation to the penis.
Teach the client to recognize signs of infection of site.	The client needs to be able to distinguish normal yellow discharge from purulent, foul smelling discharge of infection.
Teach the client that minimal bleeding is expected from circumcision site.	Excessive bleeding must be promptly identified and reported to health care provider.
Teach the client when wound is expected to be healed.	Circumcision is fully healed by well baby check-up at 2-4 weeks.

Discuss the positives and negatives of circumcision and your feelings about parents who decline circumcision.

PROS:
- Easier hygiene
- Fewer UTIs
- Decrease in risk of penile cancer
- Decreases incidence of STDs

CONS:
- Minor surgery
- Causes pain
- High risk for error if primary care provider is poorly skilled
- Circumcision can lead to infections and hemorrhage

Situation: You are called to the birthing room to assist with newborn assessment and care for a woman at 32 weeks gestation. His birth weight is 1100 grams. The infant's Apgar scores are 3 at one minute and 7 at five minutes. The infant is having nasal flaring, grunting, substernal and intercostal retractions. He is flaccid, lying in a frog-like position. The baby is covered with a thick, cheesy substance and lanugo is widely distributed over his body.

---

1. Describe the unique characteristics of a preterm infant that you may see at this birth (list 5).

   Vernix

   Lanugo

   Short soft nails

   Decreased cartilage in ears

   Translucent skin

2. Which of the assessment findings indicate that a complication may be developing?

   Nasal flaring, grunting, substernal and intercostal retractions indicate that the baby is experiencing respiratory distress. The frog-like position, vernix caseosa, and lanugo are normal assessment findings for a premature newborn at 32 weeks gestation.

3. Based on the data provided, write a nursing diagnosis for this baby.

   Either or all of the following might be used:

   Impaired Gas Exchange related to inadequate surfactant production and immature lungs

   Ineffective Breathing Pattern related to immature neurological development

   Risk for Ineffective Airway Clearance related to lack of cough/gag reflex and mucus obstructing the very narrow bronchi and trachea

4. Why is this baby at risk for Ineffective Thermoregulation?

> His low birth weight and gestational age mean that he has little glycogen stored in his liver and little brown fat available for producing heat. The preterm infant lacks subcutaneous fat to insulate his body, and his flaccid muscle tone does not allow him to take a flexed position to prevent heat loss.

5. How will maintaining a neutral thermal environment facilitate the baby's growth?

> A neutral thermal environment decreases the calories needed to maintain body temperature; the calories can then be used for growth.

6. What treatment for Impaired Gas Exchange can contribute to development of hypothermia in this baby? What can the nurse do to prevent it?

> The baby will most likely require oxygen therapy. The nurse should assure that the oxygen is warmed and humidified. The baby will, of course, be placed in an incubator with an ISC probe for temperature regulation.

Situation: Baby B., one hour old, was born at 42 weeks gestation as documented by ultrasound and LMP. He has loose skin with little subcutaneous fat. He has no lanugo and no vernix caseosa, but does have a great deal of hair on his head, as well as long fingernails. His skin is dry, cracked, and peeling. His skin, umbilical cord, and nails are meconium stained. The baby weighed 7 lbs at birth. His Apgar scores were 6 and 7 at one minute and five minutes, respectively.

1. Based on these data, what can you infer about placental functioning during the last weeks of pregnancy?

   The data shows symptoms of postmaturity (or dysmaturity) syndrome. You can infer that the placental function has deteriorated, interfering with the supply of oxygen and nutrients to the fetus.

2. What ongoing assessments are especially important for this infant, and why?

   Temperature: Because the baby has little subcutaneous fat to provide insulation, he is at risk for hypothermia.

   Respirations and lung sounds: If the baby aspirated meconium at birth, he may have respiratory distress.

   Skin color: Because the fetus undoubtedly suffered from chronic uterine hypoxia, he may be polycythemic.

   This predisposes him to hyperbilirubinemia, which is characterized by jaundice.

   Heel stick for blood glucose level; Do at birth and again in one hour. Because of a compromised nutrient supply due to the aging placenta in utero, the baby probably has poor glycogen stores, and is prone to hypoglycemia.

3. What can the nurse do to help prevent hypoglycemia? Provide rationale for your answers.

Feed the baby soon after birth and feed more frequently than usual to compensate for the poor nutrition in utero.

Keep the baby warm. Hypothermia leads to hypoglycemia because it increases the infant's metabolic rate.

Newborn who is Large for Gestational Age Answer Key

Situation: An obese, multiparous woman at 40 weeks of gestation has just given birth to a baby. After prolonged pushing in second stage, a forceps-assisted birth was necessary. The baby weighs 9 lbs 8 oz. (4318 grams). The baby has marked caput succedaneum and marked bruising about the face, head, and shoulders.

---

1. How would you characterize this baby: preterm, term, post-term, LGA, SGA, or AGA (appropriate for gestational age)?

    The baby is term (40 weeks) and LGA (large for gestational age).

2. What risk factors for LGA do you find in this situation?

    Obesity, multiparity

3. In order to plan individualized care for this baby, what information should be obtained from the mother's history?

    It is important to know what, if any, maternal condition may have caused the infant to be LGA. The nurse needs to know, especially, if the mother is diabetic, if there is Rh incompatibility between the mother and the infant, or if the parents are just large people.

4. From the history, the nurse determines that the mother is not diabetic, both the mother and infant have Rh-positive blood, and that there are many large people in both families. For this infant, what assessments should the nurse make?

    Monitor vital signs.

Assess for congenital heart defects (apical pulse, color, etc.).

Screen for hypoglycemia (heel stick) and polycythemia (hemoglobin >22 g/dL).

Assess for signs of damage to the brachial plexus or facial nerve (e.g., the newborn's arm lies limply at the side; one side of the baby's face may droop or may not move when the baby cries).

Assess for a fractured clavicle (e.g., knot or lump on clavicle, no Moro reflex or spontaneous movement of the arm on the affected side).

5. Write a psychosocial nursing diagnosis for the parents of this infant.

Risk for anxiety (about the baby's well-being) related to the appearance of the baby (e.g., bruising)

Delayed bonding related to fear of causing the infant pain

6. How is the care of this baby similar to the care of another infant of the same weight, but who is born at 42 weeks of gestation? How is it different?

Both infants would need the care given to all LGA babies (e.g., assess for birth injuries, hypoglycemia, and polycythemia). The infant at 42 weeks of gestation, however, would also need to be assessed for postmaturity syndrome, and is at higher risk for hypoglycemia and respiratory distress (secondary to meconium aspiration).

Newborn who is Small for Gestational Age Answer Key

Situation: Baby G is born at 36 weeks of gestation. He is small for gestational age due to his mother's having pregnancy-induced hypertension during pregnancy. He appears long and thin, has sparse hair, a thin cord, dry skin, and a wide-eyed look - characteristics of "asymmetric" growth restriction that begins in the second half of pregnancy.

---

1. The following nursing diagnoses and collaborative problems are identified for Baby G. Supply their etiologies.

   • Impaired Gas Exchange related to: **aspiration of meconium**.

   • Potential Complication of SGA--Hypoglycemia related to: **decreased glycogen stores secondary to inadequate in utero nutrition.**

   • Hypothermia related to: **small muscle mass and lack of subcutaneous fat**.

   • Altered Nutrition: Less than Body Requirements related to: **the increased viscosity of the blood secondary to chronic intrauterine hypoxia.**

   • Risk for Altered Tissue Perfusion (Or Potential Complication--Polycythemia) related to: **increased viscosity of the blood secondary to chronic intrauterine hypoxia.**

   • Risk for Altered Parenting related to: **separation of parents and newborn because of baby's illness.**

2. Write goals/outcomes for each of the nursing diagnoses in #1.

   Baby G is free from respiratory complications (respirations are normal in rate and character; lung sounds are clear).

   Baby G maintains a stable glucose reading (>45 mg/dL).

Baby G maintains a stable body temperature (>98 F).

Baby G takes feedings without physiologic distress and gains weight at expected rate.

Baby G has normal hemoglobin reading.

Express concerns about the baby; parents demonstrate bonding behaviors.

3. Baby G's parents express concern that he is so "skinny." They are afraid he will always be small for his age. How should the nurse respond?

Babies with asymmetric (late pregnancy) growth restriction usually "catch up" in growth if they are adequately nourished after birth.

Situation: Baby girl J.P. was born less than one hour ago. Her gestational age is 38 weeks and she is 10 lb 5 oz. J.P.'s mother was diagnosed with gestational diabetes at 26 weeks' gestation. The baby's first blood glucose reading is slightly under 40 mg/dL. J.P.'s heart rate is 120, her respirations are 80, and she is not flexing her arms and legs as newborns usually do. The mother intends to breastfeed J.P., but she has not yet attempted to do so.

1. What risk factor(s) for hypoglycemia are present in this situation?

    Maternal diabetes, LGA

2. Is the baby hypoglycemic?

    Yes.

3. What symptoms of hypoglycemia are present in this baby?

    Blood glucose <45 mg/dL, rapid respirations, and hypotonia

4. What measures are needed to treat the baby's hypoglycemia? Why?

    Promote feeding to supply glucose to provide energy and replenish stores.

    Institute measures to keep the baby warm to prevent cold stress, which increases glucose metabolism.

Organize care to minimize stresses to the baby: stress increases the metabolic rate.

Monitor for tachypnea and apnea and support respirations as needed (symptoms of hypoglycemia).

NOTE: Monitoring blood glucose levels and observing for signs of hypoglycemia would certainly be appropriate; however, they are observations, not "treatments."

5. Write three nursing diagnoses that should take priority at this time.

Consider Risk for Injury, Altered Nutrition: Less than Body Requirements, Impaired Gas Exchange, Risk for Altered Parent/Infant Attachment, and Anxiety (parental)

6. The mother attempts to breastfeed baby J.P., but the baby will not latch on and suck, even though the nurse has been present to assist the mother. What should the nurse do next?

Refer to a lactation consultant for alternate methods to support breastfeeding. However, it is vital that the infant remains well-hydrated and maintains a stable blood sugar.

7. In addition to measures to directly increase the blood glucose, how is care for baby J.P. similar to the care given to an infant who is small for gestational age?

It is extremely important to protect both infants from cold stress and to observe for respiratory distress.

Situation: E.M. is a one-day-old, full-term newborn. She weighs 7 lbs 1 oz. (3.2 kg). She is receiving phototherapy because of jaundice secondary to ABO incompatibility. E.M. is breastfeeding, but has been sleepy and is feeding poorly. She has had several loose green stools. Her skin and mucous membranes are slightly dry, skin turgor is good, and the anterior fontanel is flat. Her urine is slightly dark.

1. Why does E.M. have loose green stools?

   E.M.'s stools are green because the phototherapy causes increased bile flow and peristalsis.

2. Place a "P" beside the nursing interventions that are being done because of E.M.'s **phototherapy**. Place an "H" beside the interventions that are being done to treat the **hyperbilirubinemia**. (NOTE: Some interventions may serve **both** purposes; mark them "PH.") Provide rationale for your answers.

   PH Feed infant every 2-3 hours.

   P   Weigh all diapers.

   P   Check urine specific gravity.

   H   Maintain a neutral thermal environment and prevent cold stress.

   H   Dress infant in warm clothes and blankets when removing her from phototherapy.

   H   Observe for lethargy, high-pitched cry, absent Moro reflex, and seizures.

   P   Turn infant frequently.

3. What, if any, symptoms of Fluid Volume Deficit does E.M. have?

   Dry mucous membranes

4. How could the nurse monitor E.M. for Fluid Volume Deficit?

   Continue to check her skin turgor and fontanel.

   Weigh her diapers; urine output should be 1-3 mL/kg/hr.

5. During the past two hours, E.M. has had one wet diaper with a net weight of 4 grams. (a) How many ounces of urine per hour does this represent? (b) Is this adequate output for E.M.?

   This is equal to 4 mL in two hours, or 2 mL/hour.

   This is not adequate. Urine output should be 1-3 mL/kg/hr. Since E. M. weighs 3.2 kg, her output should be at least 3.2 mL/hour, and perhaps even as much as 9.6 mL/hour.

6. In light of the information about E.M. output, what should the nurse do?

   The baby has not been breastfeeding well, so it will probably be necessary to bottle-feed her some formula. If this improves her output, and if she shows no further signs of dehydration, intravenous therapy may not be needed.

7. What nursing diagnoses should the nurse use for E.M.? For her parents?

   For E.M., consider Fluid Volume Deficit, Risk for Altered Skin Integrity, Risk for Injury, and Ineffective Breastfeeding.

8. Provide etiologies for the following nursing diagnoses for E.M.

Fluid Volume Deficit r/t frequent loose stools and insensible water loss secondary to phototherapy, and also r/t insufficient fluid intake secondary to ineffective breastfeeding

Risk for Impaired Skin Integrity r/t frequent loose stools

Risk for Injury r/t exposure of eyes and gonads to phototherapy

Situation: J.B. is a premature, appropriate-for-gestational-age (AGA), male infant, who weighed 2 kg (4.4 lbs.) at birth. His Apgar scores were 5 and 7. J.B. is in an incubator, receiving oxygen and CPAP. He is attached to a cardiac monitor and a pulse oximeter. His respiratory rate is 68 per minute, heart rate is 150 beats per minute, and temperature is 97.4° F rectally. He has sternal retractions, nasal flaring, and expiratory grunting with his breathing. His mother wishes to breastfeed him, but he is presently being gavage fed because he is too lethargic to latch on and suck effectively.

1. List the client data in the situation.

   Premature, AGA, male, birth weight 2 kg, Apgars 5 and 7, respirations 68/minute, heart rate 150/minute, temperature 97.4° F rectally, sternal retractions, nasal flaring, expiratory grunting. Such things as "gavage feeding" and "receiving oxygen" are treatments that J. B. is receiving, not client data.

2. Place an "**R**" beside the data that represent **risk** factors for RDS. Place an "**S**" beside the data that represent **symptoms** of RDS. Place an "**N**" in the blank if it is **neither** a risk factor nor a symptom of RDS.

R	**Prematurity**
N	**AGA**
R	**Male**
S	**Apgars of 5 and 7**
S	**Respirations 68/minute**
N	**African-American**
S	**Sternal retractions, grunting, nasal flaring**
N	**Rectal temperature 97.40 F**
S	**Heart rate 150 bpm**

3. What is the relationship between J.B.'s being in the incubator and his RDS?

Of course J.B. would be in the incubator because of his prematurity and low temperature, even if he did not have RDS. However, because he has RDS, it is even more important to prevent hypothermia. Cold stress would further decrease surfactant production, leading to atelectasis. It also increases anaerobic metabolism, which is already present in RDS; and it increases the baby's metabolic rate, oxygen consumption, and glucose utilization, which are already compromised because of increased work of breathing that is present in RDS.

4. Write three nursing diagnoses that would be appropriate for J.B. State both problem and etiology.

Consider:
Impaired Gas Exchange related to inadequate lung surfactant secondary to prematurity

Altered Nutrition:
Less than Body Requirements r/t increased metabolic needs (stress and increased work of breathing)

Interrupted Breastfeeding r/t necessity for gavage feedings

Activity Intolerance r/t inadequate oxygenation and metabolic demands created by difficulty breathing

Risk for Hypothermia r/t prematurity and inadequate fat stores

1. Which of the following newborns is/are at risk for sepsis?

   Baby A, who was born at 35 weeks gestation and was large for gestational age

   Baby B, who was born at 40 weeks gestation and was large for gestational age

   Baby C, a triplet whose mother experienced gestational diabetes

   Baby D, whose mother took medications to treat infertility before he was conceived

   Baby E, who is Rh+ and whose mother is Rh-

   Baby F, who was born at 40 weeks gestation and is small for gestational age

   Baby G, whose mother uses cocaine and experienced several weeks of bleeding from mild placental separation.

   Baby H, whose mother worked in a factory until 4 weeks before the birth

   Baby I, who will be discharged home with his mother and father, who has tuberculosis

   Answer: Baby A, C, F, G, and I

2. In which of the following newborns should neonatal sepsis be suspected? (Temperatures are all axillary.)

   Baby A: Temperature 100° F, dry mucous membranes, minimal urinary output

   Baby B: Temperature 97° F, feeding poorly, lethargic, pale, and jittery

   Baby C: Temperature 98.4° F, nasal flaring and grunting with respirations, mottled, with periods of apnea

   Baby D: Temperature 96.8° F, jaundiced, feeding poorly

   Baby E: Temperature 98.2° F, diarrhea, vomiting, rash

   Answer: Baby A probably has a temperature elevation because of dehydration; fever is not a typical symptom of sepsis neonatorum. All the other babies have symptoms of sepsis.

3. Which, if any, of the babies in #2 can definitely be said to have sepsis?

   None. Their symptoms could be from other causes. It is necessary to perform diagnostic tests (e.g., blood and urine cultures, CBC, chest x-rays, and so on) in order to diagnose sepsis.

4. Which, if any, of the babies in #2 have symptoms that should be reported?

   All of them

Situation: F.J. is two days old. She is in the neonatal intensive care unit because of sepsis neonatorum. F.J. has vomiting, diarrhea and a skin rash. She has been feeding poorly and her skin turgor is poor. Her urine output is less than normal. She is receiving intravenous Ampicillin and will be tube fed to provide calories.

---

5. Based on these data, what nursing diagnoses can you make for F.J.?

   Risk for Infection Transmission (to others)

   Fluid Volume Deficit r/t inadequate intake and excessive loss secondary to diarrhea and vomiting

   Risk for Impaired Skin Integrity r/t rash and diarrhea

   Risk for Altered Nutrition: Less than Body Requirements r/t feeding poorly and vomiting (Note that risk factors for altered nutrition are present; however, there are not yet symptoms of altered nutrition. Therefore, an "actual" problem of Altered Nutrition is not appropriate.)

6. What nursing actions are needed for Risk for Infection Transmission?

   The nurse must control the nursery environment to prevent the spread of F.J.'s infection to others:
   - **Monitor and insist on strict hand washing technique for all who enter the nursery.**
   - **Wear gloves and other barriers, as appropriate.**
   - **Use aseptic technique to collect specimens for laboratory tests.**
   - **Change and clean incubators at least weekly.**
   - **Remove and sterilize wet equipment every 24 hours.**
   - **Be sure that linen, stethoscopes, etc., are not cross-used between infants.**
   - **Clean sinks and soap containers frequently (according to policy).**
   - **Be aware that it is easier to isolate an infant in an incubator than in an open radiant warmer.**
   - **Discourage visits to the nursery by unnecessary personnel and visitors.**

Newborn with Substance Withdrawal Answer Key

Situation: B.J. is 72 hours old. He was born prematurely at 32 weeks' gestation and was exposed to cocaine and heroin in utero. He is SGA, not feeding well, but sucks frantically on a pacifier. He is being fed through a nasogastric tube and regurgitates much of his feedings. His temperature is 100° F, pulse is 140, and respirations are 70 per minute. He is on an apnea monitor. B. J. has had six watery stools in the past 24 hours and has lost 10% of his birth weight. He has mild tremors when stimulated, and cries often with a high-pitched cry.

---

1. What symptoms of maternal cocaine abuse does B.J. have?

    SGA, prematurity, irritability, high-pitched cry

2. What symptoms of maternal opiate abuse does B.J. have?

    Feeding poorly, increased non-nutritive sucking, regurgitating feedings, tachypnea, fever, diarrhea, weight loss, tremors, and high-pitched cry

3. For which complications should the nurse be especially watchful?

    Respiratory distress

    Aspiration of feedings

    Seizures

    Sudden infant death syndrome (SIDS)

4. What would be important to include in teaching with B.J. mother/parent?

    Effects of drug/substance use on the infant, techniques to soothe this infant

5. Why is it important to refer B.J.'s family to social services? What other community resources would be critical for this family?

It is vital B.J. obtains support for substance abuse during pregnancy. Additionally, the nurse's role is to assess indications of parent-infant attachment as this is a high-risk setting for a newborn. The nurse will teach the mother about infant care as needed. After birth, the infant with passive addiction will likely exhibit jitteriness, irritability, emesis, diarrhea, and sleeplessness for up to sixteen weeks after birth. This increases the likelihood of stress within the home. Ongoing teaching and community support are indicated.

Ackley, B. & Ladwig, G. (2003). *Nursing diagnosis handbook* (6th ed.). St. Louis, MO: Mosby, Inc.

Centers for Disease Control and Prevention. (2005). Standards for pediatric immunization practice. *The Journal of Family Practice. 42, S17-18.*

Ferrell, M. (2003). Improving the care of women with gestational diabetes. *Journal of Maternal/Child Nursing.* 28(5), 301-5.

Kozier, B., Erb, G., Berman, A., & Burke, K. (2003). *Fundamentals of nursing concepts, process, and practice* (7th ed.). Upper Saddle River, NJ: Prentice Hall Health.

Ladewig, P.W., London, M.L., Moberly, S.M., & Olds, S.B. (2006). *Contemporary maternal-newborn nursing care* (6th ed.). Upper Saddle River, NJ: Prentice Hall.

Lowdermilk, D., I & Perry, S. (2002). Maternity nursing, 6th Ed. St. Louis, MO: Mosby, Inc.

Lowdermilk, D.L., Perry, S.E., & Bobak, I.M. (2000). *Maternity and women's health care* (7th ed.). St. Louis, MO: Mosby, Inc.

Maloni, J., Brezinski-Tomasi, J. & Johnson, L. (2001). Antepartum bed rest: Effect on the family. *Journal of Obstetrical, Gynecological and Neonatal Nurses.*

Miller-Keane (2003) *Encyclopedia and Dictionary of Medicine, Nursing, and Allied Health* (7th ed.). Philadelphia: Saunders.

Olds, S. B., London, M. L., Ladewig, P.W. & Davidson, M. R. (2004). *Maternal-newborn nursing and women's health care* (7th ed.). Upper Saddle River, NJ: Pearson Prentice Hall.

Pillitteri, A. (2003). *Maternal & child health nursing: Care of the childbearing and childrearing family* (4th ed.). Philadelphia: J.B. Lippincott Company.

Simpson, K. & Creehan, P. (2001). Perinatal nursing. *Association of Women's Health, Obstetric, and Neonatal Nurses.* Lippincott: Philadelphia, PA

Wong, D. L., Perry, S. E., Hockenbery, M. J. (2002). *Maternal child nursing Care* (2nd ed.). Mosby: St. Louis.

Youngkin, E. & Davis, M. (2004). *Women's health: A primary care clinical guide.* (3rd Ed.). New Jersey; pearson Prentice Hall.